The Interrelationship of Surgery and Radiation Therapy
in the Treatment of Cancer

Frontiers of
Radiation Therapy and Oncology

Volume 5

Editor
JEROME M. VAETH, San Francisco, Calif.

Associate Editors
JEROLD P. GREEN, ALAN F. SCHROEDER, KENNETH R. McCORMACK,
DONALD G. BAKER and MARY LOUISE MEURK

University Park Press · Baltimore · London · Tokyo

The Interrelationship of Surgery and Radiation Therapy in the Treatment of Cancer

Proceedings of the
Fifth Annual San Francisco Cancer Symposium

With 85 figures and 81 tables

San Francisco Cancer Symposium, 5th, 1969.

19 70

University Park Press · Baltimore · London · Tokyo

Originally published by S. Karger AG, Basel, Switzerland
Distributed exclusively in the United States of America and Canada by
University Park Press, Baltimore, Maryland

Library of Congress Catalog Card Number LC 77-141819
International Standard Book Number (ISBN) 0-8391-0555-X

S. Karger AG, Arnold-Böcklin-Strasse 25, CH-4000 Basel 11 (Switzerland)

Index

Foreword VII

Dedication to Dr. J. A. DEL REGATO VIII

PEREZ, C. A. (St. Louis, Mo.): Preoperative Irradiation in the Treatment of Cancer. Experimental Observations and Clinical Implications. 1

INCH, W. R.; McCREDIE, J. A. and SUTHERLAND, R. M. (London, Ont.): Effect of X-Radiation to Tumor Bed on Local Recurrence 30

BELLI, J. A. (Boston, Mass.); DICUS, G. J. and NAGLE, W. (Dallas, Tex.): Repair of Radiation Damage as a Factor in Preoperative Radiation Therapy. 40

GOLDMAN, J. L. and FRIEDMAN, W. H. (New York, N. Y.): Investigative Aspects of Preoperative Irradiation for Advanced Carcinoma of the Larynx and Laryngopharynx. 58

ROTKIN, I. D. (Chicago, Ill.): What can we Believe? Some Observations on the Design of Clinical Investigations 72

GALANTE, M.; BENAK, S., Jr. and BUSCHKE, F. (San Francisco, Calif.): Radical Preoperative Radiation Therapy in Primarily Inoperable Advanced Cancers of the Oral Cavity 93

BILLER, H. F. and OGURA, J. H. (St. Louis, Mo.): Planned Preoperative Irradiation for Laryngeal and Laryngopharyngeal Carcinoma 100

SILVERSTONE, S.M.; GOLDMAN, J. L. and RYAN, J. R. (New York, N.Y.): Combined High Dose Radiation Therapy and Surgery of Advanced Cancer of the Laryngopharynx 106

HENDRICKSON, F. R. (Chicago, Ill.): The Results of Low Dose Preoperative Radiotherapy for Advanced Carcinoma of the Larynx 123

HAMBERGER, C.-A. and MÅRTENSSON, G. (Stockholm): Carcinoma of the Paranasal Sinuses, Combined Approach 130

DOGGETT, R. L. SCOTTE, III (Sacramento, Cal.); GUERNSEY, JAMES M. and BAGSHAW, MALCOLM A. (Palo Alto, Cal.): Combined Radiation and Surgical Treatment of Carcinoma of the Thoracic Esophagus 147

ALLEN, C. V. (Portland, Ore.): High Dose Preoperative Radiation Therapy in Carcinoma of the Rectosigmoid Colon 155

ROSWIT, B.; HIGGINS, G. A.; SHIELDS, W. and KEEHN, R. J. (Bronx, N. Y.): Preoperative Radiation Therapy for Carcinoma of the Lung: Report of a National VA Controlled Study. 163

PAULSON, DONALD L. (Dallas, Tex.): The Role of Preoperative Radiation Therapy in the Surgical Management of Carcinoma in the Superior Pulmonary Sulcus 177

FLETCHER, G. H.; MONTAGUE, E. D. and WHITE, E. C. (Houston, Tex.): Preoperative
Radiation Therapy in the Management of Breast Cancer. 188
McWHIRTER, R. (Edinburgh): Simple Mastectomy and Radical Radiation Therapy in
Cancer of the Breast 198
DAO, T. L. and HSIA, T. W. (Buffalo, N. Y.): Postoperative Radiotherapy in the
Treatment of Breast Cancer 206
WHITMORE, W. F., Jr. (New York, N. Y.): Preoperative Irradiation with Cystectomy
in the Management of Bladder Cancer 231
SCHROEDER, A. F. (San Francisco, Calif.); CREWS, Q., Jr. and ROTNER, M. B. (San Diego,
Calif.): Combined Treatment of Non-Seminoma Testicular Cancer. A Follow-Up
Study 240
LONG, R. T. L. (Florence, Ala.): Recent Trends in the Management of Advanced
Ovarian Carcinoma. 251
FLETCHER, G. H.; RUTLEDGE, F. N. (Houston, Tex.) and DELCLOS, L. (Oviedo):
Adenocarcinoma of the Uterus. 262

Foreword

The dogma of surgery first and radiation therapy for postsurgical residual disease or recurrence is no longer valid. The modalities of surgery and radiation therapy are in the management of the majority of cancers complimentary to each other. This combined role of these modalities was the subject at the Fifth Annual San Francisco Cancer Symposium on October 17 and 18, 1969. There is little doubt that local recurrences are minimized by properly administered radiation therapy in cancer of the aerodigestive tract, breast, endometrium and rectum. Definite improvement in cure rates in cancers of the paranasal sinuses, laryngeopharynx and superior pulmonary sulcus have resulted from the addition of radiation therapy to surgery. The precise role of the combined modalities in the treatment of cancer of the esophagus, lung, breast, bladder, testes and ovary remains undefined. There appears to be a definite trend away from 'low dose' preoperative radiation therapy toward 'high dose' or 'radical' radiation therapy. These subjects were explored and supporting basic laboratory data correlated with the clinical information in this symposium, 'The Interrelationship of Surgery and Radiation Therapy in Treatment of Cancer'.

JEROME M. VAETH, M. D.

Director, Claire Zellerbach
Saroni Tumor Institute
of San Francisco
Mt. Zion Hospital and
Medical Center

Dedication to Dr. J. A. del Regato

The Fifth San Francisco Cancer Symposium and its proceedings are dedicated as a Festschrift to commemorate the sixtieth birthday of J. A. DEL REGATO, M. D. DR. REGATO is Director of Penrose Cancer Hospital, Colorado Springs, and co-author of probably the most authorative text on Oncology – CANCER. His dedication to teaching is exemplified by the fact that he has trained 24 of the 118 radiation therapists in the United States who are certified in Therapeutic Radiology. Many of his trainees are now chiefs of departments in medical schools and cancer centers. He is recipient of the Gold Medal of the American College of Radiology. Because of his devotion to the specialty of Radiation Therapy and cancer, we have affectionately dedicated this symposium and this volume.

Acknowledgement

The Fifth Annual San Francisco Cancer Symposium received major support from the California Division, American Cancer Society. Additional assistance was supplied by Applied Radiation Corporation and Varian Associates.

Front. Radiation Ther. Onc., vol. 5, pp. 1–29
(Karger, Basel/München/Paris/New York 1970)

Preoperative Irradiation in the Treatment of Cancer

Experimental Observations and Clinical Implications [1]

C. A. PEREZ

Division of Radiation Therapy, Mallinckrodt Institute of Radiology, Washington University School of Medicine, St. Louis, Mo.

Even though an increased understanding of tumor biology and a better description of the patterns of spread of malignant tumors have developed in recent years, and considerable refinement has taken place in both the surgical and radiotherapeutic approaches to cancer, cure rates in many instances have not reflected these advances [7, 8]. It is not surprising, therefore, that there has been renewed interest in combining two or more therapeutic procedures in an effort to increase the effectiveness of treatment. As long ago as 1914, SYMONDS mentioned the possible benefits of irradiation before surgical treatment of large, inoperable rectal tumors, using radium applications [72]. Since then, an entirely new rationale for combined radiation and surgical therapy of cancer has arisen from the development of a cellular approach to the treatment of neoplasia [54]. That is, a distinction must be drawn between preoperative irradiation that is carried out to render an inoperable tumor operable, and that which is performed in order to enhance the surgical cure rate in operable tumors. Of course, both concepts underlie the application of preoperative irradiation, but it is the latter which has been of primary concern in many of the reports that have been published evaluating preoperative irradiation in the treatment of carcinoma of the laryngo-pharynx [23, 24, 49, 62, 69], lung [5, 37], breast [6, 11, 18, 75], ovary [34, 36], esophagus [40, 61], stomach [40], colon and rectum [35, 67], endometrium [2],

[1] With support of American Cancer Society Grant T322A and USPHS (NCI) Cancer Center Grant CA10435.

urinary bladder [73, 76] and bone and soft tissues [78] and the one that has dominated our thinking in the studies discussed in this paper.

Mechanisms of Dissemination of Cancer

As pointed out by COLE *et al.* [10], there are at least four mechanisms by which malignant tumor cells are disseminated into adjacent tissues or to distant organs: (1) local spread by contiguity to tissues in areas adjacent to the tumor, (2) permeation of lymphatics, (3) vascular invasion with incorporation of cells into the systemic circulation, and (4) mechanical implantation at the time of manipulation of the tumor (fig. 1, 2). Numerous experimental observations and clinical experience showed that tumor cells may be disseminated at the time of the surgical procedure. Washings of the operative site and collections of blood from vessels draining the tumor at the time of surgery have demonstrated the presence of tumor cells [3, 41, 58, 66]. It is not uncommon to find local recurrences at the site of the suture or at the operative site after resection of a malignant tumor. Using an ingenious experimental technique, similar to that described by HAVERBACH and SMITH [22], FEDER *et al.* [14, 16] demonstrated the transfer of mouse rhabdo-

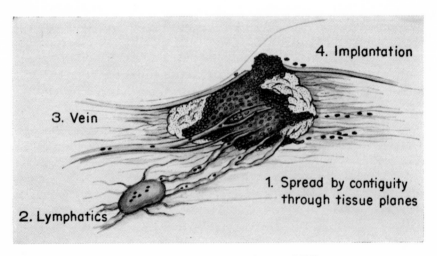

Fig. 1. Routes of spread of malignant tumors. From COLE *et al.* [10].

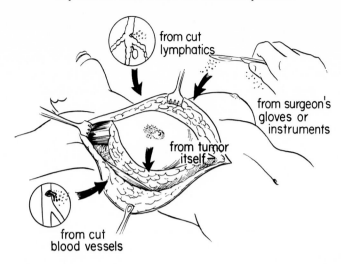

from cut
lymphatics

from surgeon's
gloves or
instruments

from tumor
itself

from cut
blood vessels

Fig. 2. Mechanisms of dissemination of tumor cells at time of surgical resection. From COLE *et al.* [10].

myosarcoma cells with a surgical needle. These observations indicate that tumor cells are able to proliferate and initiate a new tumor when they are in an adequate environment. Nevertheless, it is well known that not all of the patients in whom evidence of circulating malignant cells is found develop metastases, suggesting that there are host defense mechanisms that inactivate these cells or decrease their ability to initiate further tumor growth [10].

Rationale of Preoperative Irradiation

Since the failure to cure a malignant tumor by surgical resection may arise from the inability of the surgeon to completely remove all extensions of the lesion, or from the dissemination of cancer cells at the time of operation, it has been postulated that the administration of preoperative radiation, which will render a large fraction of the cancer cells incapable of growth, should reduce the incidence of treatment failures [54]. Ever since the demonstration that an approximately exponential relation exists between the dose of ionizing radiation administered to a population of mammalian cells and the surviving fraction of these cells [4, 12, 27, 53, 55], (fig. 3) a strong biological basis for preoperative irradiation has become evident [48]. *In vitro* and *in vivo* studies of the response of mammalian cells to ionizing radiation [77] have shown that the D_{10} – the dose that reduces the viable cell population to 10% of its initial value – generally lies between about 500 and 2,000 rads single dose for aerobic cells, and it is often smaller. It is clear, therefore, that relatively small doses of radiation, in the range of 500–2,000 rads, will inactivate the vast majority of a population of cells. (In contrast, a very much larger dose of radiation, perhaps 5,000–7,000 rads, is required for inactivation of a sufficiently large fraction of the tumor cell population to yield a high probability of cure, that is, for virtual sterilization). Furthermore, it has been shown that a fraction of the tumor cells may be anoxic [9, 26, 53, 56, 57], and since the response of the anoxic cells to irradiation is smaller and will dominate the behavior of the entire population [19], the dose necessary to obtain a cure might be even higher – sometimes so high as to cause injury to the patient's normal tissues.

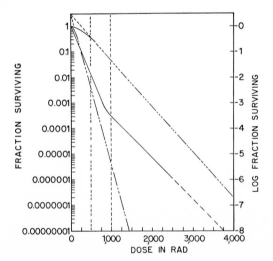

Fig. 3. Cell survival curves after irradiation. Curves A and C represent wide values reported for mammalian cells (mean lethal dose of 75 and 250 rads respectively, with extrapolation numbers of 2–3. Curve B shows the *in vivo* radiation response of the 6C3HED tumor cells as reported by POWERS and TOLMACH. From POWERS and TOLMACH [54].

   The combination of irradiation and operation has consequently been advocated in the treatment of a number of malignant tumors on the basis that the inactivation of the reproductive capacity of a larger portion of the cells by the radiation, possibly reducing the number of surviving cells by a factor of 10 or 100, or even 1,000, will inactivate a corresponding fraction of the relatively few cancer cells remaining in the irradiated region after surgical removal of the tumor mass [48, 51, 54]. This reduced viability, in turn, will decrease the probability that regrowth of the tumor will be initiated.

   An additional mechanism by which preoperative irradiation might affect the ability of residual tumor cells to initiate regrowth of a tumor lies in the effect that the radiation can have on the capacity of the host tissues to support tumor cell growth. STENSTROM, SUMMERS and VERMUND et al. [68, 71, 74] and HEWITT and BLAKE [25] have shown that irradiation of the tumor bed prior to the implantation of tumor cells will decrease significantly the number of takes as compared with unirradiated tissues. This may be the result of effects on blood vessels, lymphatics, or the stroma of connective tissue. However, our experiments have led us to conclude that it is more likely that the beneficial effect of preoperative irradiation lies in the direct killing of the tumor cells by ionizing irradiation.

   A possible effect of low dose preoperative irradiation in enhancing the development of metastases should not be ignored. YAMAMOTO [79], KAPLAN et al. [33] and others [13, 17, 42] have demonstrated an increased frequency of pulmonary metastases in mice following local low-dose irradiation of tumors. However, this has not been definitely confirmed in clinical series and the potential benefit of preoperative irradiation might well outweigh this potentially deleterious effect.

Indications for the Use of Preoperative Irradiation

It is important to identify those patients who, from either clinical or biological considerations, may be expected to benefit from preoperative irradiation. These patients include those in whom local recurrence of the tumor is likely to develop because of dissemination of tumor cells into the wound area; because microextensions of the tumor, which are clinically unrecognized, are not removed at the time of the surgical procedure, or because metastatic deposits originate from cells disseminated at the time of operation. In general, only empirical knowledge of the response to surgery of different types of tumors can provide the necessary information with which to identify these patients. It is recognized, of course, that many patients develop metastases because of malignant cell dissemination prior to the surgical procedure, and that such patients will not benefit by preoperative irradiation.

Another group of patients in whom preoperative irradiation may be of value consists of those who have such extensive tumors that initial resection is impossible because of involvement of adjacent vital structures. The preoperative administration of ionizing radiation may reduce the size of this mass and its extension, rendering the tumor resectable after partial regression. As noted above, however, the biological considerations under discussion here do not apply to this group.

The following additional groups of patients will *not* be expected to benefit from preoperative irradiation [48, 51]: (1) Those with clinically localized, easily resectable lesions which have a low probability of extending into adjacent tissues or of metastasizing. (2) Those with clinically unrecognized metastases at the time of the surgical resection of the tumor. By definition, identification of these lesions is impossible at present, though statistical analysis of clinical experience might provide a basis for assigning a patient to this group. (3) Those with lesions that can be treated successfully either by irradiation or surgery alone. The possibility of increasing the incidence of complications in this group argues strongly against administering preoperative irradiation. Clearly, a combination of clinical experience, thorough knowledge of oncology, and familiarity with the principles of cellular radiation biology are required to assess the desirability of preoperative irradiation in any particular case.

Experimental Studies

A number of experimental studies utilizing laboratory animals, mainly mice, have demonstrated benefit from preoperative irradiation in the treatment of various tumor-host systems (table I). Significant increases in cure rates were demonstrated with combinations of noncurative doses of radiation and surgical resection, as compared with operation alone. For example, POWERS and TOLMACH [54] reported beneficial results with the 6C3HED (Gardner) lymphosarcoma growing in C3H/Anf mice, the same animal tumor system that we have used for the experiments reported in this paper. The experimental methods used in that work were also employed in the present studies [43, 44, 45, 46, 47].

A tumor was produced by intradermal or subcutaneous injection of a suspension of cells into the flanks of a group of C3H/Anf mice. Tumors were palpable after several days, depending on the size of the inoculum. When tumors appeared, the animals were randomly allocated into groups which were treated with (a) 500 rads of 230 kV X-rays, (b) resection of the tumor with a wide skin flap, or (c) 500 rads immediately before resection of the tumor. A dose of 500 rads alone produced no cures, and the operation alone yielded 53% cures; the combination of 500 rads and surgery gave 85% cures. The probability of this difference in cure rate occurring by chance (X^2 test) is less than 0.001.

The 6C3HED lymphosarcoma is known to metastasize only rarely. For example, in a group of mice with advanced tumors in which microscopic sections of lungs and liver were examined, only about 5% of the animals were found to have metastatic lesions in these organs. Furthermore, unsuccessfully treated mice always presented recurrences at or near the site of the original tumor. Clearly, this particular animal tumor model system is not a good analog of most cancer patients, and is not useful for the evaluation of preoperative irradiation in preventing distant dissemination of tumor cells. Other mouse tumors, which more readily metastasize, might be more suitable. For example, SMITH and GODBEE [65] reported a significant decrease in the incidence of lung metastases after intravenous dissemination of a stem cell tumor in C57BL/6J mice, or of Cloudman S91 melanoma in DBA2/J mice, following administration of radiation therapy to the tumor-bearing area (fig. 4, 5). Nevertheless, the 6C3HED tumor has a number of attributes which render it experimentally quite useful [52].

Table I. Preoperative irradiation experimental studies in animal tumor systems

Author	Tumor	Approx. curative dose	Cure with surgery only	Preoperative irradiation dose	Cure with preoperative irradiation and surgery
NAKAYAMA *et al.*, 1963 [40]	MH$_{134}$ mouse hepatoma	Not stated	3/19 (16%)	2,000 r (2 days delay for surgery)	5/18 (28%)
AGOSTINO and NICKSON, 1960 [1]	Walker 256 carcinosarcoma	Not stated	21/100 (21%)	800 r (1 day delay for surgery)	40/100 (40%)
INCH and McCREDIE, 1963 [29]	Rat Walker 256 carcino-carcinoma	6,000 r (90% cure dose)	18/35 (51%)	2,000 r	30/34 (88%)
INCH and McCREDIE, 1963 [31]	C$_3$H mouse mammary carcinoma	6,000 r (90% cure dose)	36/63 (57%)	2,000 r (1 day delay for surgery)	40/63 (66%)
INCH and McCREDIE, 1964 [31]	C$_3$H mammary carcinoma	6,000 r (90% cure dose)	33/84 (39%)	2,000 r (6 days delay for surgery)	42/71 (59%)
POWERS, 1964 [48]	B16-melanoma	5,000 r (50% cure dose)	75/122 (62%)	1,000 r	94/115 (82%)
	KHAA	5,000 r (50% cure dose)	18/60 (30%) 19/57 (33%)	1,000 r 2,000 r	40/60 (66%) 37/46 (80%)
	KHDD	5,000 r (50% cure dose)	29/63 (46%)	1,000 r	45/67 (67%)
POWERS and TOLMACH, 1964 [54]	6C3HED lymphosarcoma	3,000 r (90% cure dose)	56/106 (53%)	500 r	99/116 (85%)
DAS GUPTA and WHITELY, 1969 [21]	Rabbit Vx-2 carcinoma	5,000 r	0/45 (limited resection)	1,000 r	18/20 (1st week) (90%) 16/20 (2nd week) (80%)

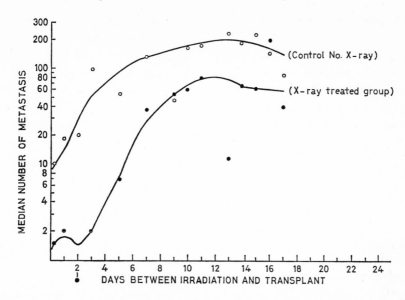

Fig. 4. Lung metastases resulting from intravenous injection of stem-cell tumor in C57BL/6J mice, with and without irradiation of the tumor with a single dose of 700 to 1,000 rads. Figure 3–2 in Smith and Godbee [65].

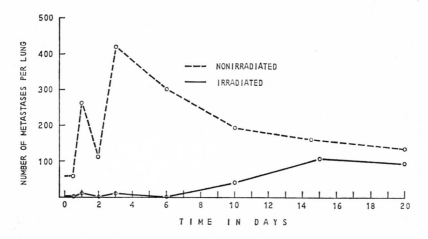

Fig. 5. Lung metastases resulting from the intravenous dissemination of Cloudman S-91 Melanoma in DBA2/J mice with and without prior *in vivo* irradiation of the tumor with a single dose of 1,200 rads. Figure 3–6 in Smith and Godbee [65].

Once the value of preoperative irradiation was demonstrated, a number of problems which we have to face in clinical situations had to be dealt with. This included optimization of the X-ray dose, the time interval between irradiation and surgery, and the fractionation schedule for the irradiation. In addition, it was necessary to consider adjuvant chemotherapy, the possibility of utilizing post-operative irradiation, and the healing of the surgical incision.

Optimal Dose of Radiation

It is evident that in administering radiation prior to a surgical procedure, consideration must be given not only to the regression of the tumor and to the number of malignant cells that one expects to inactivate, but also to the technical difficulties that might be added to the operation, and to possible interference with the healing processes necessary for preservation of anatomical and physiological integrity. Optimization of dose depends on several factors: (1) the number of cells that are to be inactivated, (2) the response of those cells to irradiation, (3) the number of viable cells required to cause recurrence of the tumor, (4) the radiation sensitivity of the normal tissues involved in the healing process. While estimates of these parameters can be made from previous work with this or other systems, combining the estimates so as to obtain maximal benefit with minimal trauma is not likely to yield a value for the optimal dose in which we can have much confidence. Direct observation with the tumor system can provide a more meaningful dose estimate.

A group of 400 mice was inoculated with the 6C3HED lymphosarcoma. When the tumor became palpable, the animals were randomly allocated into 4 groups which were treated with a single dose of 500, 1,000 or 2,000 rads. The fourth group received no irradiation. Surgical resection of the tumor was performed immediately after irradiation. The results show that with increasing doses there was a progressive improvement in the cure rate, from 20% with surgery alone, to up to 85% with 2,000 rads (fig. 6). In a second experiment, 260 mice rendered 'immunologically incompetent' by treatment with 300 rads whole body irradiation and oral hydrocortisone before receiving the tumor cell transplant,

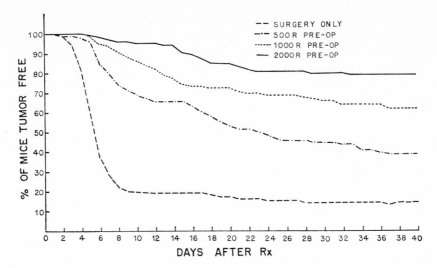

Fig. 6. Effect of preoperative irradiation on the cure of 6C3HED Gardner lymphosarcoma in normal C3H mice. The percent of mice free of overt tumors is plotted as a function of time, for various doses of preoperative radiation [47].

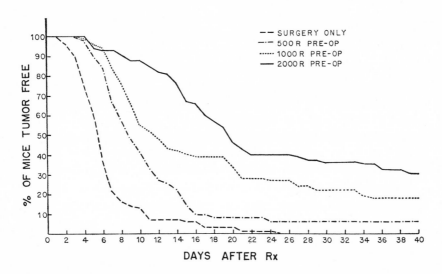

Fig. 7. Effect of preoperative irradiation on the cure of 6C3HED lymphosarcoma in C3H mice rendered immunologically 'incompetent' with 300 rads whole body irradiation and hydrocortisone in the drinking water [47].

were then treated with the same dose as in the previous experiment. The cure rate was 3 to 5 times lower (an immune reaction has been shown to play an important role in the cure of these mice). However, though the cure was markedly affected by the disturbance to the immune response, the benefit of increasing doses of pre-operative irradiation was still evident (fig. 7). This finding would indicate that, from the point of view of therapeutic success, the higher the dose of irradiation the more benefit, as expected, because more cells are killed. Similar results were reported by SLOAN et al. (63) in a mammary carcinoma transplanted in the hind leg of C3H mice. Of course, limitation must set in at higher doses as discussed above (the objective of these studies was not to cure mice by radiation therapy). From the clinical view point, HENDRICKSON and LIEBNER [23] reported no difference in results with fractionated preoperative doses of 2,000 or 5,000 rads administered to randomly selected patients with advanced supraglottic laryngeal cancer.

Optimal Time for Operation

Differences in the proliferation kinetics of various normal and tumor cells requires consideration of the optimal time for the surgical resection of the tumor following irradiation. From the point of view of regrowth of the surviving tumor cells, a minimum interval should prove to be best. For example, with the fast growing tumor used in these experiments, the longer the period of time between the irradiation and the operation, the greater the tumor growth and consequent spread. Table II shows that the repopulation of a larger fraction of surviving cells after the lower doses results in a higher incidence of large, inoperable tumors after 7 days.

If inoperable tumors are excluded, our experiments with the 6C3HED tumor demonstrate no significant improvement in the cure rates with doses over 1,000 rads, if the operating is performed immediately rather than after 1, 3 or 7 days following irradiation (fig. 8). Experiments reported by FEDER and BLAIR [14], involving the transplantation of a rhabdomyosarcoma growing in C3H mice 1, 7 or 14 days following administration of 2,000 rads showed no significant difference in the transplantability of the tumor cells

Table II. Preoperation irradiation in a C3H mouse lymphosarcoma; delay between irradiation and surgery and incidence of inoperability

Dose of radiation	Time of surgery after irradiation			
(rad)	1 day	3 days	7 days	%
500	0/56	0/60	56/60	93
1,000	0/55	0/57	18/57	31
2,000	0/57	0/57	7/65	12
3,000	0/56	0/58	10/59	17
4,000	0/53	0/57	6/58	11

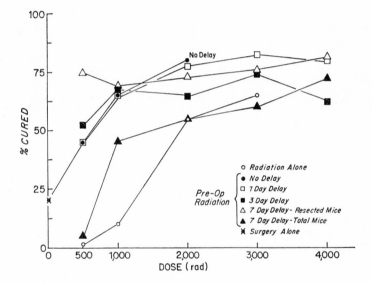

Fig. 8. Comparative cure rates of C3H mice with 6C3HED lymphosarcoma. Best results are obtained with preoperative doses of more than 1,000 rads followed by surgery immediately or one day after irradiation. Delay of 3 or 7 days resulted in higher inoperability rate, decreasing the cure rates for the entire population of mice in those groups. Cure rates for X-rays alone is included for comparison [47].

after these time intervals. (They found some difference after a 3-week delay, but because of factors associated with the increasing age of the tumors, they questioned the validity of this result.) INCH and McCREDIE [31], investigating the effect of a single dose of 2,000 rads prior to surgical resection of a transplanted spontaneous mammary carcinoma in C3H mice, found that a delay of 6 days between irradiation and operation was more effective in reducing local recurrence than was a 1- or 12-day delay. SLOAN et al. [63] reported lower cure rates of a C3H mammary carcinoma in mice when resection was delayed for 6 days after varying doses of radiation in comparison with immediate removal of the tumor following irradiation.

In human tumors, which comparatively grow slowly, it might be desirable to allow time for the tumor to regress before performing surgery. With such delay, a second preoperative dose of radiation immediately prior to the operation might even be considered. Another indirect potential benefit of a delay between preoperative irradiation and operation derives from the fact that some patients who are free of clinically evident dissemination of tumor at the time of irradiation might develop metastases by the time of evaluation for the surgical procedure. They might well be spared a fruitless surgical procedure [48].

Fractionation of Dose

Another clinical factor which has to be considered is the fractionation of the radiation dose, and the overall period of time in which the treatment is delivered. Fractionation allows both recovery from sublethal damage and repopulation of cells to take place between doses [12]. Particularly in rapidly growing neoplasms this applies to the tumor as well, where it is not desirable as it is in the normal tissues. The effects of fractionated irradiation in the reoxygenation of hypoxic tumor cells [32, 70] is not a pertinent consideration in preoperative irradiation. The bulk of the tumor with the central anoxic component should be completely removed surgically. Optimization of fractionation is a particularly good example of a problem that may be easier to deal with empirically than on the basis of calculations from measured parameters.

Experiments were carried out with mice allocated into several groups. One group was treated by surgical resection of the tumor only. Other groups received doses of 500, 1,000, 2,000, 3,000, 4,000 or 5,000 rads to the tumor in a single treatment, in three equal fractions over a period of 5 days, or in six equal fractions over a period of 12 days. Surgical resection of the tumor was performed immediately after the single doses or after the last treatment in the fractionated schedules. Surgery alone yielded 37% cures (11 out of 30 mice). The addition of single or fractionated preoperative doses of X-rays enhanced tumor control significantly (fig. 9). A single preoperative dose of 500 rads produced a 75% cure rate and 1,000 rads, 80%; the fractionation of 500 rads into 3 fractions reduced the cure rate to 41%; and of the mice treated with 1,000 rads divided in 6 fractions only 4 were operable because of marked growth of the tumor by the completion of the course of irradiation: only 1 of the 4 animals was cured. Otherwise, the fractionation of doses greater than 1,000 rads into 3 or 6 treatments yielded cure rates comparable to those obtained with single doses. It is evident

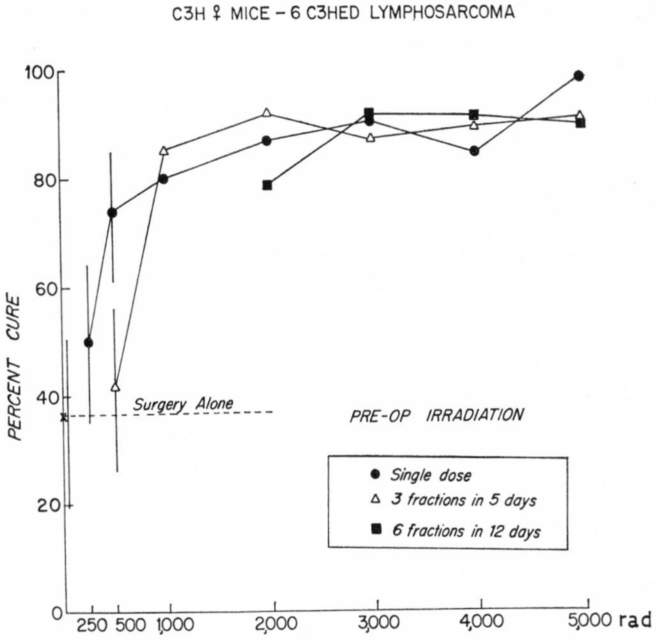

C3H ♀ MICE – 6 C3HED LYMPHOSARCOMA

Fig. 9. Comparison of cure rates with single or fractionated doses of X-irradiation in C3H mice with Gardner lymphosarcoma. Below 1,000 rads single doses more effective than fractionated doses. With larger amounts of radiation no difference in cure rate is noted (P = 0.05). Vertical bars indicate 95% confidence limits.

that small single doses (500 and 1,000 rads) were equally as effective as larger fractionated doses [45]. Using a C3H rhabdomyosarcoma in mice and various doses of radiation, FEDER *et al.* [15] reported a similar decrease in effectiveness of small dose preoperative irradiation when this was fractionated. This was more striking with lower doses (total of 2,000 rads given in one, two or five fractions in a period of 1 week).

Preoperative Irradiation and Adjuvant Chemotherapy

The use of chemical or chemotherapeutic agents at the time of surgical resection of a tumor and/or following surgery has been proposed on essentially the same basis that preoperative irradiation has been advocated, i.e., in an effort to eliminate the reproductive capacity of the malignant cells so that the number of locally or distantly disseminated cells that remain viable is diminished [28, 30, 59, 64]. Such inactivation can result in a significant decrease of both local recurrences and distant metastases. In fact, because tumor cells that might have migrated out of the irradiation field prior to treatment would be subject to inactivation by the chemotherapeutic agent, drugs might have certain advantages over radiation as an adjuvant to surgery. Of course, they also present certain disadvantages, such as toxicity to the body's cells renewal systems which often limits drug therapy.

Although possible effects on distant metastases do not play a role with the 6C3HED tumor system, we undertook an evaluation of the effect of combined drug, irradiation, and surgical therapy on this tumor. Prior to the surgical resection of the tumor, groups of animals received single intraperitoneal injections of approximately 1/10 of the LD50 of any one of 4 drugs (table III). Another group of animals received single preoperative doses of X-rays to the tumor-bearing flank (500, 1,000, 2,000 or 3,000 rads), in addition to the drug.

Preoperative administration of any of the 4 drugs significantly increased the cure level (50% with nitrogen mustard or cyclophosphamide and 78% with vincristine or vinblastine) above that achieved with drugs only or with surgery alone (20%). The combined preoperative administration of a chemotherapeutic agent and X-radiation prior to the resection of the tumor produced further increases in the cure rates with doses of 1,000 and 2,000 rads, as compared with preoperative irradiation (fig. 10). Since the sensitivity of the 6C3HED cells to chemotherapeutic agents has not been investigated, quantitative interpretation of the results of this experiment is difficult. The picture is further complicated by the immunological response that the C3H mouse exhibits to this tumor [38, 52], which plays a part in effecting cures with relatively small doses of X-rays. However, it is postulated that the enhanced effectiveness of the combination of these 3 methods of treatment lies in the inactivation by X-rays of a large fraction of the cells in the irradiated area, the inactivation by drugs of those tumor cells which have already disseminated outside the operative field, and the surgical removal of those cells localized in the primary lesion [44].

Table III. Preoperative irradiation and chemotherapy in the cure of a 6C3HED lymphosarcoma (chemotherapeutic agents)

Drug	LD_{50} (mg/kg)	Dose per mouse (mg)
Nitrogen mustard (mechlorethamine HC1)	4	8
Cyclophosphamide	50	1
Vincristine sulfate	2	4
Vinblastine sulfate	3	6
Single intraperitoneal injection		

Possibilities of Adjuvant Immunotherapy

There is little doubt that immunological phenomena play an important role in tumor biology. A growing body of evidence indicates that numerous tumors in experimental animals, whether elicited by carcinogens or viruses, possess antigenic activity capable of provoking immunological responses [60], and similar phenomena have been demonstrated experimentally in spontaneous and transplanted animal tumors [20]. Preliminary data from our

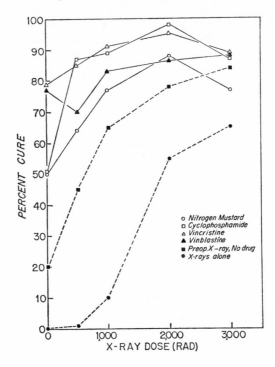

Fig. 10. Cure of 6C3HED lymphosarcoma with a combination of preoperative irradiation, drugs and surgical resection. Percentage cure is plotted as a function of X-ray dose for each of the chemotherapeutic agents tested. Results with X-rays alone or preoperative irradiation and resection without drugs are included for comparison [44].

laboratory, using anti-6C3HED lymphosarcoma serum produced in rabbits, have shown the effectiveness of this anti-serum in preventing the development of tumors in animals injected with 10^4, 10^5, or 10^6 lymphosarcoma cells [43]. Preliminary results of an experiment with a small group of mice treated with pre-operative irradiation and intraperitoneal injection of 1 ml of anti-tumor serum followed by resection of the tumor, demonstrated an appreciable improvement in cure rates over those obtained with surgical resection of the tumor alone, or with a combination of preoperative irradiation and surgery (table IV). As in the case of chemotherapy (which is also a systemic treatment), the added effectiveness of the combined treatment may be explained by inactivation of cells lurking outside of the irradiated tissues, and/or by the added inactivation by the antitumor serum of cells surviving the irradiation. The administration of anti-lymphocyte serum or anti-KHT tumor serum to mice failed to produce any decrease in the number of lymphosarcoma takes, strongly suggesting the specificity of the antibodies against the 6C3HED lymphosarcoma. Additional experiments are being performed at the present time, and will be reported later.

Table IV. 6C3HED lymphosarcoma in C3H mice, effect of adjuvant intraperitoneal anti-tumor serum injection (cure rates)

Dose (rad)	No surgery				Yes surgery			
	Normal rabbit serum	%	Anti-tumor serum	%	Normal rabbit serum	%	Anti-tumor serum	%
0	0/12		0/13		9/19	47	11/13	85
500	0/18		2/16	13	6/16	38	15/15	100
1,000	8/16	50	6/12	50	12/18	67	14/15	93

Comparison with Postoperative Irradiation

As stated by Moss, whenever postoperative irradiation is indicated, preoperative irradiation should have been given [39]. The effects of postoperative irradiation should be similar to those of preoperative irradiation, except for the basic difference that irradiation after manipulation and surgical resection of the tumor have occurred will not affect those cells that were disseminated in the latter procedures.

Postoperative irradiation has been used 'prophylactically' in an effort to decrease the incidence of local recurrences (as in carcinoma of the breast following radical mastectomy). It has also been used when the surgeon has reason to believe that the tumor has not been completely removed, or that cells have been disseminated in the operative field. Finally, it has been applied when the tumor has been found to be incompletely resectable.

In a series of experiments designed to compare the effectiveness of pre- and postoperative irradiation in controlling the 6C3HED lymphosarcoma in mice, we found that at doses below 3,000 rads, preoperative irradiation significantly increased the cure rate, in comparison with postoperative irradiation (fig. 11). At higher doses, both methods were equally efficacious in enhancing the surgical cure rates. We have attempted to explain these results on 2 bases: (1) The tumor bed may be altered by the surgical procedure, such that there is a decreased oxygen tension in the operative wound as a consequence of capillary injury. This would result in a decreased response of the tumor cells in the animals irradiated after operation. (2) Tumor cells may be disseminated into the marginal tissues outside of the irradiated field. While preoperative irradiation would greatly affect the reproductive capacity of disseminated cells, postoperative irradiation cannot reach these cells unless the marginal tissues received a cancerocidal dose. The high incidence of local failures (at the suture line) in mice treated by surgery alone, or by combined surgery and post-

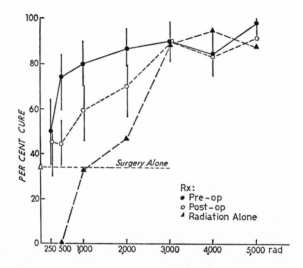

Fig. 11. Comparison of pre- and postoperative irradiation in the cure of 6C3HED lymphosarcoma. The percentage cure is plotted as a function of dose. The curves demonstrate significantly different results after preoperative and postoperative irradiation, up to 2,000 rads; postoperative irradiation is not as effective at low doses. The cure rate by surgery alone, from previous experiments, is included for comparison (P = 0.05). Vertical bars indicate 95% confidence limits [46].

operative irradiation, as compared with those treated preoperatively (fig. 12), would support either of these two hypotheses. Furthermore, we cannot discard the theoretical possibility of an immunological derangement at the operative site due to a block of cellular or circulating antibodies which would thereby be unable to inactivate those viable tumor cells which escaped radiation inactivation.

Healing of Normal Tissues

While the mechanism of wound healing has not been completely elucidated, there is reason to believe that cell proliferation in the wounded region originates from the immediately adjacent tissues

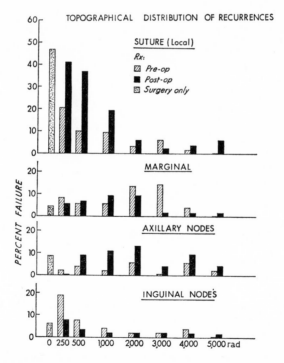

Fig. 12. Histograms showing the topographical distribution of recurrences. Local failures are markedly greater in mice treated by operation alone or with low doses of postoperative irradiation (below 2,000 rads). Recurrences in other sites are not appreciably different for any of the methods of treatment compared [46].

[48]. X-irradiation must affect the normal cells as well as the tumor cells that lie in the radiation field; hence, preoperative irradiation would be expected to interfere with the processes by which the surgical wound heals. Although cure of the malignancy may be the primary consideration in the treatment of a patient, the healing of the wound and the preservation of anatomical and physiological integrity are also of fundamental importance.

POWERS *et al.* [50], demonstrated that increasing doses of irradiation above 1,000 rads produced progressive delays in the healing of surgical wounds in the skin of mice. Confirmation of this finding can be seen in many of our experiments with preoperative irradiation in the cure of the 6C3HED lymphosarcoma.

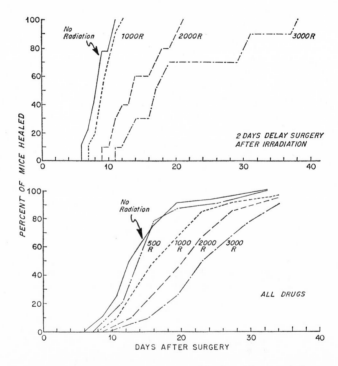

Fig. 13. Effect of preoperative irradiation on wound healing. The cumulative percentage of mice healed is plotted as a function of time for each dose of radiation. The upper panel shows previous results obtained with X-rays alone [50]. The lower panel shows combined results with four drugs and X-rays. The delay in wound healing from the drug treatments is equivalent to that caused by about 1,200 rads of X-rays [44].

The combination of cytotoxic drugs and irradiation, used in certain of the experiments reported previously, produced a greater delay in healing than does irradiation alone, as would be expected from the increased cell killing. The concentration of the chemotherapeutic agents employed produced an added delay in the healing of normal tissues, equivalent to that brought about by irradiation with 1,200 rads (fig. 13). Interestingly, a similar degree of enhancement was observed in the response of the tumor.

It has been postulated that postoperative irradiation may be more detrimental to the healing process than is preoperative irradiation, because the former is necessarily delivered to all of the cells proliferating in the area of the wound, while the latter will not reach those cells which migrate into the wound area subsequent to surgery. Nevertheless, our experiments have failed to show any significant difference between pre- and postoperative irradiation with respect to a delay in wound healing (fig. 14).

Conclusions

Though the usefulness of preoperative irradiation has not been definitely demonstrated in clinical practice, a significant number of animal experiments strongly suggest that this therapeutic approach may provide a means of increasing the expectation of curing certain malignant tumors. Doses of irradiation of the order of 20–30% of the therapeutic dose, followed by surgical removal of the tumor, have been shown to contribute significantly to the control of malignant growths in numerous experimental animals. Several clinical studies have been reported showing some benefit from preoperative irradiation but, unfortunately, most of them did not include adequate control series.

Treatment of very small, localized lesions, which are highly curable, will probably not benefit from combined therapy. Likewise, if the disease has been disseminated, but the spread is clinically inapparent at the time of the definitive therapy, no significant benefit may be expected by any local adjuvant treatment. Tumors most likely to benefit from this combined treatment would be those that have some local extension into adjacent structures, and have not systemically disseminated at the time of

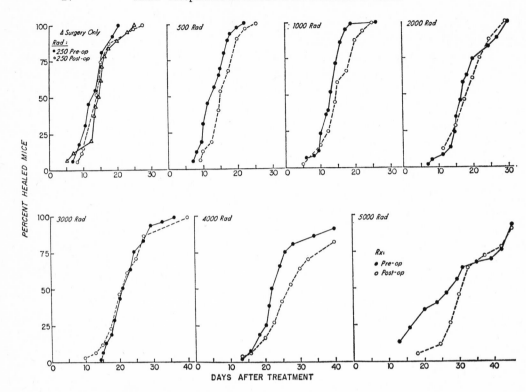

Fig. 14. Effect of pre- and post-surgical irradiation on wound healing with higher doses of radiation. No statistically significant difference in pre- or postoperatively treated animals was observed [46].

operation. However, it is possible that the additional administration of chemotherapeutic agents (or perhaps in the future, of specific anti-tumor serum) may inactivate those systemically disseminated tumor cells which cannot be affected by the localized irradiation or the resection of the tumor, with resulting increase in cure rates.

The prolonged duration of treatment that has often been selected with adjuvant preoperative therapy has engendered criticism by some surgeons. This delay may be obviated by compact courses of low-dose preoperative irradiation, followed immediately by resection of the tumor. This should diminish technical difficulties at the time of the operation, and interference with the healing mechanism.

High doses of irradiation, combined with radical operations, usually carry a considerable morbidity and, sometimes higher, surgical mortality, but there is no evidence that low-dose irradiation, combined with surgical treatment, presents such hazards. If effective, this therapy should be readily accepted by the surgeon and it would be, in fact, the treatment of choice.

Direct extrapolation from experimental observations to clinical situations cannot be made. It is obvious that well-designed, randomized clinical trials must be carried out in patients in order to properly define the indications and the benefits of preoperative irradiation. Otherwise, its effectiveness may never be clearly elucidated. Furthermore, those factors which may alter the effects of preoperative irradiation as demonstrated in animal tumor systems must be tested in clinical situations in an effort to obtain optimal results.

References

1. AGOSTINO, E. and NICKSON, J.J.: Preoperative X-ray therapy in a simulated colon carcinoma in the rat. Radiology 74: 816–819 (1960).
2. ARNESON, A. N.: An evaluation of the use of radiation in the treatment of endometrial cancer. Bull. N. Y. Acad. Med. 29: 395–410 (1953).
3. ARONS, M. S.; SMITH, R., R. and MYERS, M. H.: Significance of cancer cells in operative wounds. Cancer 14: 1,041–1,044 (1961).
4. BERRY, R. J. and ANDREWS, J. R.: Quantitative studies of radiation effects on cell reproductive capacity in mammalian transplantable Tumor system in vivo. Ann. N. Y. Acad. Sci. 95: 1,001–1,008 (1961).
5. BLOEDORN, F. G.; COWLEY, R. A.; CUCCIA, C. A., and MERCADO, R., Jr.: Combined therapy: irradiation and surgery in the treatment of bronchogenic carcinoma. Amer. J. Roentgenol. 85: 875–885 (1961).
6. BORGSTROM, S. and LINDGREN, M.: Preoperative roentgen therapy of cancer of the breast. Acta radiol., Stockh. 58: 9–16 (1962).
7. CADY, B.: Preoperative radiation. Surg. Gynec. Obstet. 126: 851–865 and 1,091–1,105 (1968).
8. Cancer Facts and Figures (American Cancer Society, New York, 1969).
9. CLIFTON, K. H.; BRIGGS, R. C., and STONE, H. B.: Quantitative radiosensitivity studies of solid carcinomas in vivo: methodology and effect of anoxia. J. Nat. Cancer Inst. 36: 965–974 (1966).
10. COLE, W. H.; MCDONALD, G. O.; ROBERTS, S. S., and SOUTHWICK, H. W.: Dissemination of cancer: Prevention and therapy (Appleton-Century-Crofts, New York 1961).
11. DELARUE, N. C.; ASH, C. L.; PETERS, V., and FIELDEN, R.: Preoperative irradiation in management of locally advanced breast cancer. Arch. Surg. 91: 136–154 (1965).
12. ELKIND, M. M. and SUTTON, H.: Radiation responses of mammalian cells grown in culture: repair of X-ray damage in surviving Chinese hamster cells. Radiat. Res. 13: 556–563 (1960).

13. Essen, C. F. von and Kaplan, H. S.: Further studies on metastasis of a transplantable mouse mammary carcinoma after roentgen irradiation. J. Nat. Cancer Inst. *12:* 883–892 (1952).
14. Feder, B. H. and Blair, P. B.: Preoperative irradiation evaluation by a simple experimental model. Radiology *83:* 111–119 (1964).
15. Feder, B. H.; Blair, P. B., and Close, P.: Fractionation in preoperative irradiation. Radiology *84:* 447–451 (1965).
16. Feder, B. H.; Skorneck, A. B.; Green, H. W., and Blair, P. B.: Simple experimental model for measuring effectiveness of preoperative irradiation. Radiology *80:* 286–287 (1963).
17. Fisher, B. and Collins, V.: A discussion of basic aspects of preoperative irradiation; in Rush, Jr. and Greenlaw's Cancer therapy by integrated radiation and operation, pp. 28–33 (Thomas, Springfield 1968).
18. Fletcher, G. H.; Montague, E., and White, E. C.: Evaluation of preoperative irradiation for carcinoma of the breast. Proc. 5th Nat. Cancer Conf. (Lippincott, Philadelphia 1964).
19. Gray, L. H.: Radiobiologic basis of oxygen as modifying factor in radiation therapy. Amer. J. Roentgenol. *85:* 803–815 (1961).
20. Green, N. N.; Anthony, H. M.; Baldwin, R. W., and Westrop, J. W.: An immunological approach to cancer, pp. 173–188 (Butterworths, London 1967).
21. Gupta, T. K. Das and Whitely, H. W., Jr.: Role of preoperative irradiation in simulated colon cancer. Arch. Surg. *99:* 141–148 (1969).
22. Haverback, C. Z. and Smith, R. R.: Transplantation of tumor by suture thread and its prevention: experimental study. Cancer *12:* 1,029–1,042 (1959).
23. Hendrickson, F. R. and Liebner, E.: Results of preoperative radiotherapy for supraglottic larynx cancer. Amer. Otol. Rhino. Laryngol. *77:* 222–230 (1968).
24. Henschke, U. K.; Frazell, E. L.; Hilaris, B. S.; Nickson, J. J.; Tollefsen, H. R., and Strong, E. W.: Local recurrences after radical neck dissection with and without preoperative X-ray therapy. Radiology *82:* 331–332 (1964).
25. Hewitt, H. B. and Blake, E. R.: The growth of transplanted murine tumors in preirradiated sites. Brit. J. Cancer *22:* 808–824 (1968).
26. Hewitt, H. B.; Chan, D. P-S., and Blake, E. R.: Survival curves for clonogenic cells of a murine keratinizing squamous carcinoma irradiated *in vivo* or under hypoxic conditions. Int. J. Radiat. Biol. *12:* 535–549 (1967).
27. Hewitt, H. B. and Wilson, C. W.: Survival curves for tumor cells irradiated *in vivo.* Ann. N. Y. Acad. Sci. *95:* 818–827 (1961).
28. Hoye, R. C. and Smith, R. R.: The effectiveness of small amounts of preoperative irradiation in preventing the growth of tumor cells disseminated at surgery. Cancer *14:* 284–295 (1961).
29. Inch, W. R. and McCredie, J. A.: Effect of a small dose of X-radiation on local recurrences of tumors in rats and mice. Cancer *16:* 594–598 (1963).
30. Inch, W. R. and McCredie, J. A.: Effect of wound irrigation with nitrogen mustard to clorpactin XCB on local recurrence of rat and mouse tumors. Cancer *16:* 599–602 (1963).
31. Inch, W. R. and McCredie, J. A.: Preoperative use of a single dose of X-rays. Arch. Surg. *89:* 398–406 (1964).
32. Kallman, R. F.: Repopulation and reoxygenation as factors contributing to the effectiveness of fractionated radiotherapy. Frontiers of Radiation Therapy and Oncol. vol. 3, pp. 97–108 (Karger Basel/New York 1968).
33. Kaplan, H. S. and Murphy, E. D.: The effect of local roentgen irradiation on the biological behavior of a transplantable mouse carcinoma-I; increased frequency of pulmonary metastases. J. Nat. Cancer Inst. *9:* 407–413 (1949).

34. KOTTMEIER, H. L.: Modern trends in the treatment of patients with semi-malignant and malignant ovarian tumors. Symposium on carcinoma of the uterine cervix, endometrium and ovary, pp. 296 (Year Book, Chicago 1962).

35. LEAMING, R. H.; STEARNS, M. W., and DEDDISH, R. R.: Preoperative irradiation on rectal carcinoma. Radiology 77: 257–263 (1961).

36. LONG, R. T. and SALA, J. M.: Radical pelvic surgery combined with radiotherapy in the treatment of locally advanced ovarian carcinoma. Surg. Gynec. Obstet. 117: 201–204 (1963).

37. MALLAMS, J. T.; PAULSON, D. L.; COLLIER, R. E.; and SHAW, R. R.: Presurgical irradiation in bronchogenic carcinoma, superior sulcus type. Radiology 82: 1,050-1,054 (1964).

38. MITCHISON, N. A.: Studies on the immunological response to foreign tumor transplants in the mouse. I. The role of lymph node cells in conferring immunity by adoptive transfer. J. exp. Med. 102: 157–177 (1955).

39. MOSS, W. T.: Therapeutic radiology, rationale, technique results, p. 32 (Mosby, St. Louis 1965).

40. NAKAYAMA, K. et al.: Concentrated preoperative irradiation therapy. Arch. Surg., Chicago 87: 1,003–1,008 (1963).

41. NASH, S. C.; MALMGREN, R. A.; HUME, R., and SMITH, R. R.: Tumor cells in postoperative wound drainage. Cancer 15: 221–226 (1962).

42. OLCH, P. D.; STLVENSON, J. K., and HARKINS, H. N.: Further studies of the effect of local sublethal tumor irradiation on the development of distant metastases. Surg. Forum 11: 61–63 (1960).

43. PEREZ, C. A. and HUNT, J.: Passive immunity as an adjuvant to surgical and irradiation therapy of a mouse lymphosarcoma (to be published).

44. PEREZ, C. A. and OLSON, J.: Preoperative irradiation and chemotherapy in the cure of a mouse lymphosarcoma. Radiology 92: 136–142 (1969).

45. PEREZ, C. A. and OLSON, J.: Preoperative irradiation. Experimental studies on fractionation. Presented at the 53rd meeting, Radiological Society of North America, Chicago, December, 1968.

46. PEREZ, C. A. and OLSON, J.: Preoperative vs. postoperative irradiation. Experimental observations in a mouse lymphosarcoma. Amer. J. Roentgenol. (Accepted for publication.)

47. PEREZ, C. A. and POWERS, W. E.: Studies on optimal dose of preoperative irradiation and time for surgery in the cure of a mouse lymphosarcoma. Radiology 89: 116–122 (1967).

48. POWERS, W. E.: Theoretic basis and experimental evidence supporting preoperative radiation therapy. Proc. 5th Nat. Cancer Conf., pp. 461–467 (Lippincott, Philadelphia 1964).

49. POWERS, W. E. and OGURA, J. H.: Preoperative irradiation in head and neck cancer surgery. Arch. Otolaryng. 81: 153–160 (1965).

50. POWERS, W. E.; OGURA, J. H., and PALMER, L. A.: Radiation therapy and wound healing delay – Animals and man. Presented at the November, 1966 meeting of the Radiological Society of North America, Chicago. Radiology 89: 112–115 (1967).

51. POWERS, W. E. and PALMER, L. A.: Biologic basis of preoperative radiation treatment. Amer. J. Roentgenol. 102: 176–192 (1968).

52. POWERS, W. E.; PALMER, L. A., and TOLMACH, L. J.: Cellular sensitivity and tumor curability. Nat. Cancer Inst. Monogr. 24: 169–185 (1965).

53. POWERS, W. E. and TOLMACH, L. J.: Multicomponent X-ray survival curve for mouse lymphosarcoma cells irradiated in vivo. Nature, Lond. 197: 710–711 (1963).

54. POWERS, W. E. and TOLMACH, L. J.: Preoperative radiation therapy, biological basis and experimental investigations. Nature, Lond. 201: 272–273 (1964).

55. Puck, T. T. and Marcus, P. I.: Actions of X-rays on mammalian cells. J. exp. Med. *103:* 653–666 (1956).

56. Putten, L. M. Van and Kallman, R. F.: Effect of pre-irradiation on the ratio of oxygenated and anoxic cells in a transplanted mouse tumor. 3rd int. Congr. Rad. Res. Abstracts, Cortina (Abstr. 910) (1966).

57. Reinhold, H. S.: Quantitative evaluation of the radiosensitivity of cells of a transplantable rhabdomyosarcoma in the rat. Europ. J. Cancer *2:* 33–42 (1966).

58. Roberts, S.; Jonasson, O.; Long, L.; McGrew, E. A.; McGrath, R., and Cole, W. H.: Relationship of cancer cells in circulating blood to operation. Cancer *15:* 332–340 (1962).

59. Sako, K.; Marchetta, F. C.; Badillo, J., and Burke, E.: Results of cytologic studies of wound washings and use of local cytotoxic agent in head and neck surgery. Amer. J. Surg. *102:* 818–822 (1961).

60. Schwartz, R. S.: Are immunosuppressive anti-cancer drugs self-defeating? Cancer Res. *28:* 1,452–1,454 (1968).

61. Seymour, E. Q. and Pettit, H. S.: Preoperative X-ray therapy in cancer of the esophagus. Radiol. *85:* 952–955 (1965).

62. Silverstone, S. M.; Goldman, J. L., and Rosin, H. D.: Combined therapy irradiation and surgery for advanced cancer of the laryngopharynx. Amer. J. Roentgenol. *90:* 1,023–1,031 (1963).

63. Sloan, K. W.; Bloedorn, F. G., and McCredy, W. A.: Combined surgical and X-ray treatment of isotransplants of a mouse mammary adenocarcinoma. Radiology *90:* 366–367 (1968).

64. Smith, R. R. and Gehan, E. A.: Effect of formaldehyde wound wash on development of local wound recurrences. J. Nat. Cancer Inst. *23:* 1,339–1,345 (1959).

65. Smith, R. R. and Godbee, G. A.: Alteration of tumor cell implantability by preoperative irradiation; in Rush, Jr. and Greenlaw Cancer therapy by integrated radiation and operation, pp. 20–27 (Thomas, Springfield 1968).

66. Smith, R. R.; Ketcham, A. A.; Malmgren, R. A., and Chu, E. W.: Cancer cell wound contamination associated with surgical therapy of carcinoma of cervix. Cancer *16:* 1,100–1,104 (1963).

67. Stearns, M. W., Jr.: Preoperative irradiation of cancer of the rectum. Proc. 5th Nat. Cancer Conf., pp. 489–493 (Lippincott, Philadelphia 1964).

68. Stenstrom, K. W.; Vermund, H.; Mosser, D. G., and Marvin, J. F.: Effects of roentgen irradiation on the tumor bed. I. The inhibiting action of local pre-transplantation roentgen irradiation (1,500 r_a) on the growth of mouse mammary carcinoma. Radiat. Res. *2:* 180–191 (1955).

69. Strong, E. W.; Henschke, U. K.; Nickson, J. J.; Frazell, E. L.; Tollefsen, H. R., and Hilaris, B. S.: Preoperative X-ray therapy as an adjunct to radical neck dissection. Cancer *19:* 1,509–1,516 (1966).

70. Suit, H. D. and Maeda, M.: Hyperbaric oxygen and radiobiology of a C3H mouse carcinoma. J. Nat. Cancer Inst. *39:* 639–652 (1967).

71. Summers, W. C.; Clifton, N. H., and Vermund, H.: X-irradiation to the tumor bed. Radiol. *82:* 691–702 (1964).

72. Symonds, C. J.: Cancer of the rectum; excision after application of radium. Proc. roy. Soc. Med., Clin. Sect. *7:* 153 (1913–14).

73. Veenema, R. J.; Buttman, R.; Uson, A. C.; Sagerman, R. H.; Dean, A. L., and Ciardullo, L.: Combined radiotherapy, surgery and chemotherapy in carcinoma of the bladder. Cancer *20:* 1,879–1,885 (1967).

74. Vermund, H.; Stenstrom, K. W.; Mosser, D. G., and Loken, M. K.: Effects of roentgen irradiation on the tumor bed. III. The different inhibiting action on the growth of mouse mammary carcinoma resulting from pre- or post-transplantation irradiation. Radiat. Res. *8:* 22–31 (1958).

75. WHITE, E. C.; FLETCHER, G. H., and CLARK, R. L.: Surgical experience with preoperative irradiation for carcinoma of the breast. Ann. Surg. *115:* 948–956 (1962).
76. WHITMORE, W. F., Jr. *et al.*: Preoperative irradiation with cystectomy in the management of bladder cancer. Amer. J. Roentgenol. *102:* 570–576 (1968).
77. WHITMORE, G. F. and TILL, J. E.: Quantitation of cellular radiobiological responses. Ann. Rev. Nucl. Sci. *14:* 347–374 (1964).
78. WINDEYER, B.; DISCHE, S., and MANSFIELD, C. M.: The place of radiotherapy in the management of the soft tissues. Clin. Radiol. *17:* 32–40 (1966).
79. YAMAMOTO, T.: An experimental study on the effect of X-ray on metastasis of malignant tumor, especially in bones. Jap. J. Obstet. Gynec. *19:* 388–392 (1936).

Author's address: Dr. CARLOS A. PEREZ, Mallinckrodt Institute of Radiology, 510 South Kingshighway, *St. Louis, MO 63110* (USA).

Front. Radiation Ther. Onc., vol. 5, pp. 30–39
(Karger, Basel/München/Paris/New York 1970)

Effect of X-Radiation to Tumor
Bed on Local Recurrence[1]

W. R. INCH, J. A. McCREDIE, and R. M. SUTHERLAND

Ontario Cancer Treatment and Research Foundation, London Clinic and the Departments of
Therapeutic Radiology and of Surgery, University of Western Ontario, London, Ont.

Local cancer recurrence is due to growth of malignant tissue left
at the site of excision of a tumor or not destroyed by radiotherapy
or chemicals; occasionally it may follow excision from contamination of the surface of the tissues with cancer cells during the
taking of a biopsy. Ionizing radiation has been given interstitially,
by contact or by teletherapy before or after operation to reduce
local recurrence. Conventionally fractionated irradiation given
preoperatively has been used extensively in patients with locally
advanced tumors; the treatment is given over 3 to 4 weeks and
delays excision. There has been considerable interest in the use of
a concentrated course of radiotherapy immediately prior to
operation. We have studied the effect of a single large dose of
X-rays on local recurrence using syngeneic tumors in mice.

GRAY et al. [2] showed that hypoxic cells that are exposed to
X-rays are damaged less than those that are well oxygenated. Since
the vessels in tumors are poorly developed and innervated, tumor
oxygenation is largely dependent on flow in the surrounding
normal tissues. KRUUV et al. [4] found that isoproterenol, chlor-
promazine, norepinephrine and amyl nitrite decreased tumor
blood flow and oxygenation and that inhalation of 95% oxygen
(O_2) plus 5% carbon dioxide (CO_2) at atmospheric pressure
caused an increase. DU SAULT [1] and INCH et al. [3] found that
breathing the gas mixture during radiotherapy increased the rate

[1] This investigation was supported by the Ontario Cancer Treatment and Research
Foundation, Grant No. 151.

of cure of mammary tumors in mice. We have continued these studies to find if there is an optimum time to inhale 5% CO_2 and 95% O_2 before radiotherapy.

Methods

Small pieces of the spontaneous C3H/HeJ mammary carcinoma were implanted by trocar into the dorsal subcutaneous tissues of one hundred 10 to 12-week-old female offspring. Single tumors became palpable at 13 to 16 days and none regressed. At a size of about 1 cm³, the syngeneic transplants were excised and the site of excision was irrigated with 100 ml of saline (0.9 g NaCl/100 ml). The first 40 ml was collected, centrifuged and examined using the Papanicolaou staining technique for the presence of cancer cells. The incisions were closed and animals were kept for 100 days and observed for local recurrence. Serial sections of the tumor bed of representative animals were made after excision and examined for the presence of tumor.

A single biologically large dose of X-rays, 2,000 rads, was given to the tumor, 1.0 ± 0.2 cm³, and its vascular bed, 1, 6 or 12 days before operation or to the operative site 1 day after excision. A control group was given the same dose of X-rays to normal tissues cephalic to the tumor 1 day before excision. The dose of X-rays was given through parallel opposed fields, 1.5×2 cm, covering the tumor and 0.3 mm of the vascular bed, using a precision microradiotherapy technique. Positioning was carried out using a back-field localizer and beam direction was checked regularly by radiographs. Animals were kept for 100 days and observed for local recurrence.

A further experiment was performed to find the effect on local recurrence of inhaling normobaric 100% O_2 containing amyl nitrite or 95% O_2 plus 5% CO_2 before and during X-irradiation. Amyl nitrite, 0.3 ml, was nebulized over 5 sec and inhaled for 4 min before starting X-irradiation. Control animals inhaled 100% O_2. Inhalation of 95% O_2 plus 5% CO_2 was started 0.5 or 12 min before and during X-irradiation. Control animals inhaled air, 100% O_2 for 0.5 or 12 min or hyperbaric, 4 atmospheres absolute, 100% O_2 for 4 min before and during X-irradiation. The dose of X-rays, 4,200 rads, was given through parallel opposed fields in two equal fractions separated by 4 days. Animals were kept for 100 days and observed for local recurrence. Survivors were killed and autopsied.

Results

Syngeneic transplants of the spontaneous C3H tumor that appeared within 60 days of implantation grew rapidly and a high proportion were fixed to the deep fascia by processes of tumor extending through the poorly developed capsule (fig. 1a). The remainder appeared between 60 and 120 days, grew more slowly, had a smooth surface without processes infiltrating the normal tissues and none were fixed (fig. 1b). After excision of the tumors, residual malignant tissue was found in histologic sections of the vascular beds of many of the fast growing tumors and none of those that were slow growing (fig. 2).

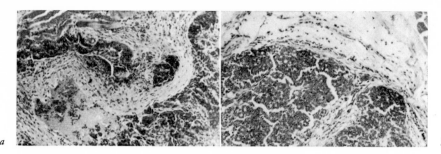

a *b*

Fig. 1. Surfaces of 'slow' and 'fast' growing C3H syngeneic transplants (H. and E. ×180).

The fast growing tumors had a higher incidence of clumps of cancer cells in the fluid used to irrigate the incisions, and a higher incidence of local recurrence. The slow growing tumors had a low incidence of clumps and of local recurrence (fig. 3).

At 50 days, irradiation of the tumor and its vascular bed 1 day before excision or to the vascular bed 1 day after excision reduced local recurrence compared with control animals (table I). By 100 days only preoperative irradiation caused a significant reduction, 34% compared with 43% for controls. When the irradiation was given 1, 6 or 12 days before operation local recurrence at 50 and 100 days was least in animals treated at 6 days, 32% and 41%, compared with the control group given irradiation to normal tissues 1 day before excision which was 51% and 61% (table II).

At 50 days local recurrence in animals that inhaled normobaric 100% O_2 with 0.3 ml amyl nitrite was increased compared to the control group that inhaled 100% O_2. By 100 days nearly all animals given amyl nitrite had developed recurrence while the incidence was only 28% in the control group that inhaled oxygen (table III).

Tumors in animals that inhaled 95% O_2 plus 5% CO_2 or 100% O_2 at 1 or 4 atmospheres before and during X-ray therapy regressed at the same rate, could not be measured after 20 days and began to recur at about 30 days. Cure based on absence of local recurrence at 100 days was least in the control group, 36%, and about 60% in the groups breathing normobaric 95% O_2 plus

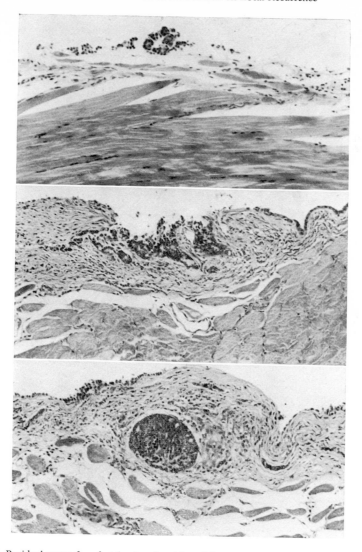

Fig. 2. Residual tumor found at the site of excision of fast growing C3H syngeneic transplants (H. and E. ×180).

5% CO_2 for 12 min, 100% O_2 for one-half or 12 min, or hyperbaric 100% O_2 for 4 min before and during X-irradiation (table IV). Cure was highest, 77%, in the group inhaling the gas mixture for one-half minute before and during treatment.

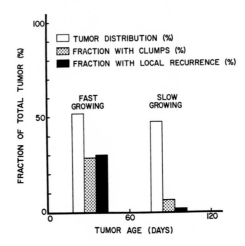

Fig. 3. Fast growing C3H syngeneic tumors had higher incidence of clumps of cancer cells in washings from incisions and of local recurrence than those that grew slowly.

Table I. Local recurrence of syngeneic tumor in C3H/HeJ mice after a single dose (2,000 rads) of X-rays one day before or after excision

Group	No. mice	Mean tumor weight (g)	Local recurrence (%) 50 days	100 days
To tumor 24 hours before excision	63	0.8±0.1[1]	8 (<0.01)[2]	34 (<0.05)
To operative site 24 hours after excision	57	1.0±0.1	14 (<0.05)	45 (>0.05)
To normal tissues on day of excision	63	1.0±0.1	25	43

[1] Standard error of mean.
[2] Probability of difference between groups using Chi-square test.

Discussion

The clumps of cancer cells found in the washings from the incisions were the result of division of tumor processes during excision. Tumor recurrence was due to growth of cells in the residual processes following excision of rapidly growing tumors; implantation of the clumps of cancer cells was probably not

Table II. Local recurrence of syngeneic C3H/HeJ mice after single dose (2,000 radr) X-rays, 1, 6 or 12 days before excision

Group	No. mice	Local recurrence (%)	
		50 days	100 days
1 day	86	40 (<0.05)[1]	51 (<0.05)
6 days	71	32 (<0.03)	41 (<0.02)
12 days	71	47 (>0.05)	52 (>0.05)
Control 1 day	84	51	61

[1] Probability of difference between groups using Chi-square test.

Table III. Local recurrence of syngeneic tumor in C3H/HeJ mice after local X-irradiation (4,200 rads) given while animal inhaled normobaric 100% O_2 with amyl nitrite

Group	No. mice	Tumor size (cm³)	Local recurrence (%)	
			50 days	100 days
100% O_2+amyl nitrite+X-rays	49	0.6±0.2	78 (<0.01)[1]	98 (<0.01)
100% O_2+X-rays	43	0.6±0.2	14	24
100% O_2+amyl nitrite	16	0.6±0.2	100	100

[1] Probability of difference between groups using Chi-square test.

important. When radiotherapy is given before operation the peripheral portion of the tumor which is responsible for local recurrence is well oxygenated and is damaged most by treatment. It is interesting that the effect of radiotherapy increased for several days after a single dose of X-rays. This suggests that in addition to the immediate effect of X-rays there is continuing damage, probably mainly through its effect on the tumor bed. Postoperative treatment to the site of excision was less effective because the operative procedure interfered with blood and lymphatic supply,

Table IV. Effect of inhaling 100% O_2 or 95% O_2 plus 5% CO_2 before and during X-irradiation on cure of the C3H syngeneic transplanted tumor

Group No.	Gas inhaled before X-rays (minutes)	No. mice	Cure (%)[1]	Significance (p value)[2]
1.	Air (12)	30	36	
2.	95% O_2+5% CO_2 (0.5)	26	77	2 vs 1<0.01
3.	95% O_2+5% CO_2 (12)	28	57	3 vs 1<0.05 3 vs 2<0.06
4.	100% O_2 (0.5)	23	61	4 vs 1<0.05 4 vs 2<0.08
5.	100% O_2 (12)	27	59	5 vs 1<0.05 5 vs 2<0.07
6.	100% O_2, 4 Atms. Abs. (5)	24	63	6 vs 1<0.05 6 vs 2<0.09

[1] Mice were considered to be 'cured' when there was no tumor at the site of the primary at 100 days.

[2] Probability of difference between groups using Chi-square test.

through release of products of tissue injury and repair, and possibly by the introduction of infection (fig. 4).

Care must be taken in applying to patients the results of investigations using animals. The dose of 2,000 rads used in this study induced a moist reaction in the skin and temporary epilation and was probably the largest that could safely be used. In patients the 'safe dose' is probably less and depends on the tissue involved and the presence of sensitive organs. It is of interest that NAKAYAMA [6] gave the same dose, 2,000 rads in one treatment or in less than two weeks to patients with carcinoma of the esophagus, breast and rectum without severe reactions. It is unlikely that a dose of 500 rads, suggested by POWERS and TOLMACH [8] based on results using a lymphosarcoma and NIAS [7] will be effective against cells in a carcinoma.

Inhalation of amyl nitrite in 100% O_2 produced a rapid and marked decrease in blood flow to the tumor and an increased flow

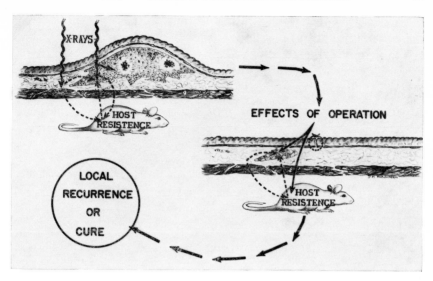

Fig. 4. Effects of preoperative X-rays on a tumor and its vascular bed.

in adjacent normal tissues. This agrees with our previous finding that some vasodilators affect the well innervated vascular bed of normal tissues by relaxing the resistance arterioles, shunting blood from the tumor and lowering the oxygen tension.

Inhalation of 95% O_2 plus 5% CO_2 for several minutes before and during X-ray therapy was shown by Du Sault [1] and confirmed by Inch et al. [3] to decrease local recurrence of the spontaneous C3H/HeJ tumor and its syngeneic transplant. Kruuv et al. [5] showed that tumor blood flow and oxygenation decreased when the animals inhaled this mixture for a long time. Results based on cure of the syngeneic C3H transplant support these data and suggest that there is an optimum time to inhale the gases before irradiation. The time may be different for humans and could be determined by inserting a platinum oxygen electrode into a tumor and measuring the oxygen diffusion current over a period of 12 min.

Another way that tumor oxygenation can be improved is inherent in the fractionation of conventional radiotherapy. Rubin and Casarett [9] have suggested that a fractionated dose of X-rays causes super-vascularization of a tumor and improves oxygenation. Supervascularization is interpreted not as an increase in total numbers of vessels but a relative increase due to tumor cell destruction and removal. Improvement in oxygenation by the methods described may be less important when the X-ray dose is fractionated and this question is now being examined.

Summary

Syngeneic transplants of the C3H mammary carcinoma in mice that appeared early, grew rapidly, developed processes of cancer cells extending into surrounding normal tissues and many recurred locally following excision. Tumors that appeared late, grew slowly, did not develop processes and few recurred. A single biologically large dose, 2,000 rads, of X-rays given to this tumor and its vascular bed 6 days before excision reduced local recurrence; it was less effective if given 1 or 12 days before excision or 1 day after excision. Inhalation of amyl nitrite in 100% O_2 before giving local irradiation to the transplant increased local tumor recurrence, probably by decreasing tumor blood flow and oxygenation. Tumor cure was higher when the animals inhaled 95% O_2 plus 5% CO_2 for one-half minute before and during X-ray therapy, than following inhalation of the mixture for 12 min, normobaric 100% O_2 for one-half or 12 min, or hyperbaric (4 atmospheres absolute) 100% O_2 for 5 min before and during X-ray therapy. This suggests that there is an optimum time to inhale this gas mixture before X-irradiation.

Acknowledgements

The authors wish to thank Mrs. M. ALDERSON, Mrs. E. EDMUNDSON and Mr. E. STROUDE for assistance during the investigation.

References

1. DU SAULT, L. A.: The effect of oxygen on the response of spontaneous tumors in mice to radiotherapy. Brit. J. Radiol. *36:* 740–754 (1963).
2. GRAY, L. H.; CONGER, A. D.; EBERT, M.; HORNSEY, S., and SCOTT, O. C. A.: Concentration of oxygen dissolved in tissue at time of irradiation as factor in radiotherapy. Brit. J. Radiol. *26:* 638–648 (1953).
3. INCH, W. R.; MCCREDIE, J. A., and KRUUV, J.: Effect of breathing 5% carbon dioxide and 95% oxygen at atmospheric pressure on tumour radiocurability. Acta Radiol. *4:* 17–25 (1966).
4. KRUUV, J.; INCH, W. R., and MCCREDIE, J. A.: Blood flow and oxygenation of tumors in mice. I. Effects of breathing gases containing carbon dioxide at atmospheric pressure. Cancer *20:* 51–59 (1967).
5. KRUUV, J.; INCH, W. R., and MCCREDIE, J. A.: Blood flow and oxygenation of tumors in mice. III. Effects of breathing amyl nitrite in oxygen on radiosensitivity of the C3H tumor. Cancer *20:* 66–70 (1967).
6. NAKAYAMA, K.: Preoperative irradiation in the treatment of patients with carcinoma of the esophagus and of some other sites. Clin. Radiol. *15:* 232–241 (1964).

7. NIAS, A. H. W.: Radiobiological aspects of preoperative irradiation. Brit. J. Radiol. *40:* 166–169 (1967).

8. POWERS, W. E. and TOLMACH, L. J.: A multicomponent X-ray survival curve for mouse lymphosarcoma cells irradiated *in vivo*. Nature, Lond. *197:* 710–711 (1963).

9. RUBIN, P. and CASARETT, G. W.: Chapter 25; in Clinical Radiation Pathology, vol 2, 1st ed., pp. 954–959 (Saunders, Philadelphia 1968).

Authors' address: Dr. W. RODGER INCH, Dr. JOHN A. McCREDIE, and Dr. ROBERT M. SUTHERLAND, Radiobiology Section, The Ontario Cancer Treatment and Research Foundation, London Clinic, Victoria Hospital, *London, Ont.* (Canada).

Front. Radiation Ther. Onc., vol. 5, pp. 40–57
(Karger, Basel/München/Paris/New York 1970)

Repair of Radiation Damage as a Factor in Preoperative Radiation Therapy

J. A. BELLI, G. J. DICUS and W. NAGLE

Department of Radiotherapy, Harvard Medical School, Boston, Mass. and Department of
Radiology, The University of Texas Southwestern Medical School at Dallas, Dallas, Tex.[1]

Introduction

The goal of preoperative radiation therapy is to reduce the probability that viable tumor cells are present within the treated volume at the time of surgery. The realization of this goal is dependent upon the elapsed time between the completion of radiation therapy and the surgical proceedure, the post-irradiation growth of tumor cells, and the repair capability of tumor cells with regard to radiation damage during and after radiation. We consider that the capacity of tumor cells to repair radiation damage is of primary importance, and will, in large measure, determine the success of a course of preoperative radiation therapy. We inquire, therefore, whether study of the radiation and recovery responses of normal and tumor cells under a variety of environmental conditions can provide sufficient insight into appropriate ways to improve the likelihood of successful preoperative radiation therapy. Our purpose will be to review our studies which bear upon these considerations. We will define some of the conditions under which radiation damage is repaired, the survival characteristics of tumor cells subjected to various schemes of fractionated irradiation, the repair capacity of hypoxic tumor cells after reoxygenation, and some aspects of the characteristics of potentially lethal damage repair by tumor and normal cells.

[1] This work was supported by PHS grants CA-08162, 5T1-CA-5136 and CA-11264 and American Cancer Society grant T-461. During a portion of this work, J. A. B. held PHS career development award, 1-K3-CA-16,925 (1965–1968).

Methods

The experiments which we will review have been accomplished with the following cell systems: (1) The P-388 lymphoma growing in DBA/2J mice as an ascites tumor; and (2) Chinese hamster female lung fibroblasts in culture.

Our methods with these systems have been described [1–4]. The serial cell dilution methods first reported by HEWITT [10] and HEWITT and WILSON [11] were used to estimate cell viability of P-388 tumor cells irradiated and assayed *in vivo*.

The Chinese hamster sublines (V79-103A and V-753; the parent line was kindly supplied to us by Dr. M. M. ELKIND, Brookhaven National Laboratory, New York, USA) were maintained in Eagle's minimal essential medium supplemented with glutamine, NCTC-109 (4%), penicillin, streptomycin, Eagle's non-essential amino acids, and fetal calf serum (15%). Maintained in this medium (FS-15) at 37°C in a humidified atmosphere of 3% CO_2, cells grew with a doubling time of approximately 9 h. Survival was assessed by the ability of cells to form macroscopic colonies growing attached to glass or plastic. Except where noted, our techniques are standard single cell plating methods as originally described by PUCK and MARCUS [12] and modified in our laboratory.

Results and Discussion

1. P-388 Tumor Cells *in vivo*

Following a standard intraperitoneal innoculum of 10^6 cells, P-388 tumor cells grew with a doubling time of approximately 12 h. As tumor growth proceeded, ascitic fluid was elaborated by the host and the tumor cell population became hypoxic. The single-dose radiation response of this tumor as a function of tumor age has been determined *in vivo* [1, 2]. The changes in survival curve parameters during tumor growth indicate that a sizable fraction of the tumor cell population is hypoxic from the fourth through seventh post-transplantation days. Figure 1 shows survival curves for 1-day and 6-day tumors. The differences in slopes are obvious, and there is a significant difference in extrapolation numbers. Whatever else these survival curve changes mean, one of the important factors influencing tumor cell response was decreased intraperitoneal oxygen tension as the tumor cell population increased and ascitic fluid was elaborated by the host.

Having demonstrated that this tumor cell system shows aerobic or hypoxic response depending upon its stage of growth, we now ask the question: Is repair capacity dependent on tumor age, and, by implication, the state of oxygenation of the tumor cell population? To provide an answer to this question, 1-day and 6-day tumors were irradiated with two doses separated by variable intervals. Survival resulting from the two doses was related to that observed with the total dose delivered in one exposure and the consequent recovery factors plotted against time between doses. Figure 2 shows the results of these experiments. The following points are important: (1) Initial repair of sublethal damage is evident in tumors of both ages. (2) The rate of initial repair appears to be slower in 6-day (hypoxic) tumors. (3) Initial repair reached a maximum 6 h after the conditioning dose in both tumors. (4) With one-day (aerobic) tumors, minimum survival was seen at 9 h followed by a second maximum at 12 h. (5) In the hypoxic condition, however, this minimum appeared to persist through 12 h. (6) The maximum recovery factor for 1-day (approximately 16) and 6-day tumors (approximately 4) was in about the same ratio as the extrapolation numbers of 1-day and 6-day tumors [5.3].

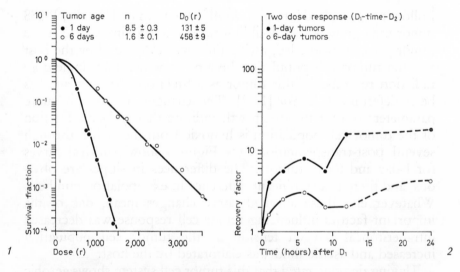

Fig. 1. Single dose survival for P-388 tumors *in vivo*. Survival fraction determined by serial dilution assay *in vivo* in DBA/2J mice. Courtesy of BELLI, BONTE and DICUS [2].

Fig. 2. Two dose response of P-388 tumors *in vivo*. Cells were allowed to remain in the animal between doses. For one day tumors $D_1 = D_2 = 500$ R; for 6-day tumors, $D_1 = D_2 = 1500$ R. Recovery factor is the survival for two doses relative to that for the total dose in one exposure. Courtesy of BELLI, BONTE and DICUS [2].

These data, therefore, clearly demonstrate that mammalian tumor cells can repair sublethal radiation damage *in vivo*. This ability appears to be present regardless of whether tumors are aerobic or hypoxic at the time of the first dose. The observed difference in the initial rates of repair may be due to several factors, but it is our conclusion that dominant among these is the hypoxic state. Thus, aerobic cells may demonstrate increased radiation response, but have a larger capacity for sublethal damage repair. Hypoxic cells, on the other hand, while demonstrating decreased radiation response, have impaired capacity for damage repair.

One of the major consequences of fractionated radiation therapy, in addition to cell killing, is reoxygenation [15–17]. As tumor volume decreases and sensitive cells are killed, the remaining tumor cell population becomes progressively better oxygenated. In the face of such environmental shifts, it becomes important to inquire whether cells damaged in the hypoxic state, and subsequently becoming aerobic, retain the capacity for sublethal damage repair. The data shown in figure 3 and figure 4 bear on this consideration. In figure 3, 6-day P-388 tumors were irradiated *in vivo* and, immediately after irradiation, transferred to new hosts in a cell concentration equal to that of 1-day tumors (3.5×10^6 cells). As a function of time after this retransplantation a second dose was delivered and tumor cells assayed for viability. It is clear that damage registered in the hypoxic state is rapidly repaired when cells become aerobic. The relative survival for a fractionation interval of 12 h after retransplantation is approximately 65 times that observed when the second dose is delivered immediately after transfer. Figure 4 shows the results of a similar experiment with the difference that the retransplantation was delayed for three hours. The closed circles show the two-dose recovery for 6-day tumor cells allowed to remain hypoxic between exposures. The open circles trace the survivals observed when damaged hypoxic cells are transfered to new hosts 3 h following the first dose. It is of interest to note that the sequence of survival fluctuations is very close to that of 1-day tumors, but displaced to the right by 3 h. The hypoxic state, therefore, does not impair the capacity for additional sublethal damage repair when the damaged cell becomes reoxygenated. These results are pertinent to the response of tu-

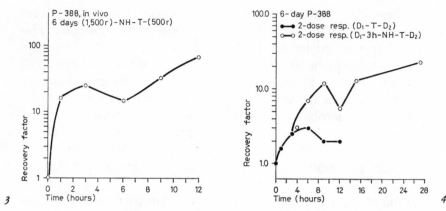

Fig. 3. Recovery response of 6-day tumor cells after a first dose of 1500 R and transplantation immediately into new hosts at a cell concentration equal to that of a one-day tumor (3.5×10^6 cells). The second dose (500 R) was given these animals at times shown by data points. Courtesy of BELLI, BONTE and DICUS [2].

Fig. 4. Recovery response of 6-day tumor cells after a first dose of 1500 R and transplantation into new hosts 3 h later. The second dose (500 R) was given these animals at times shown by the open circles. The closed circles trace the two dose response for 6-day tumor cells allowed to remain in the original host. In the latter case, $D_1 = D_2 = 1500$ R.

mors during fractionated radiotherapy. For example, it is not unlikely that tumor cells may go through repeated cycles of hypoxic damage, reoxygenation, repair and retransfer to the hypoxic fraction.

We now turn to the consideration of whether mammalian cells are able to sustain and repair repeated episodes of radiation damage. Implicit in this consideration is the question: Do survival curve parameters of cells surviving a given fractionation scheme depend upon the time and dose relationship chosen? When one starts with a predominately hypoxic tumor cell population, it may be expected that survival curve parameters will depend upon fractionation schemes because of changes in the proportion of hypoxic cells, changes in population composition, and tumor cell growth. To study these points, survival curves were determined for 6-day P-388 tumor cells after zero, 1, 2, 3, 4 or 5 fractions separated by 6, 9 or 12 h. The fractionation intervals were chosen to correspond with the initial peak and persistant minimum in the two-dose response. Figure 5 shows the variation in extrapolation number (n), D_0 and D_Q as a function of the *total* number of exposures, e.g. the parameters shown for one exposure are those resulting from single dose survival curves; those for six exposures are for cells surviving five fractions separated by 6, 9 or 12 h, etc. These data are summarized in table I. In general, D_0 values were independent of prior fractionation. Changes in extrapolation number and D_0 are always in the same direction. For all fractionation intervals a peak in the D_Q and extrapolation number occurs. For intervals of 6 h, this is seen for cells surviving four fractions of 900 R each; for 9-hour intervals, after three fractions of 1125 R. Whether the peak in extrapolation number and D_Q observed after 5 fractions of 750 R separated by 12 h would have been followed by a fall had the number of fractions been increased is not known.

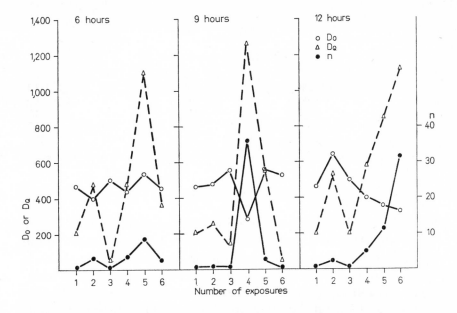

Fig. 5. Relationship between fractionated exposure and survival curve parameters. D_0, D_Q and extrapolation number (n) are plotted against *total* number of exposures including that for survival response. Times indicated refer to fractionation interval. Cells were allowed to remain in the animal for entire course. Data are for 6-day tumor cells.

Table I. Survival curve parameters as a function of fractionation interval and number of fractions

No. of fractions	Fraction size (R)	D_O (R)	D_Q (R)	n
		Six-hour intervals		
1	—	458	200	1.6
2	1500	394	469	3.3
3	1500	500	50	1.1
4	1125	431	475	3.2
5	900	535	1100	8.2
6	750	450	360	2.2
No. of fractions	Fraction size (R)	D_O (R)	D_Q (R)	n
		Nine-hour intervals		
1	—	458	200	1.6
2	1500	476	252	1.7
3	1500	556	140	1.2
4	1125	275	1260	36.0
5	900	546	550	2.8
6	750	525	40	1.04
No. of fractions	Fraction size (R)	D_O (R)	D_Q (R)	n
		Twelve-hour intervals		
1	—	458	200	1.6
2	1500	640	530	2.3
3	1500	500	200	1.4
4	1125	397	575	4.7
5	900	356	850	11.7
6	750	325	1125	31.5

For 6- and 9-hour fractionation intervals, we conclude that these peaks are associated with changes in the age-density-distribution of the surviving population and minor improvements in the oxygenation of surviving cells within the peritoneal cavity. The reciprocal relationship between D_o on the one hand and extrapolation number and D_Q on the other for 12-hour fractionation intervals is taken as a more secure demonstration that, as the number of fractions increase, a larger proportion of the remaining population becomes better oxygenated (demonstrated by the fall in D_o) with consequent changes in age-density-distribution and age-response-function (as demonstrated by the increase in extrapolation number and D_Q). Because the D_0 value decreased by a factor of two between 1 and 5 fractions, a reasonable assumption is that substantial improvement in the oxygenation of surviving cells had occurred during fractionation.

Up to this point we have demonstrated that mammalian tumor cells irradiated and assayed for reproductive survival *in vivo* have substantial capacity for sublethal damage repair under a variety of fractionation schemes under hypoxic conditions. These results have direct bearing upon the efficacy of preoperative radiation therapy. It is apparent that the success of this combined approach to the management of human cancer must take into account the amount of radiation damage repair by the tumor cell population during therapy and in the interval between the completion of therapy and surgery.

Whether the interval between completion of radiation therapy and surgery is important with regard to repair of radiation damage can be determined by the study of survival in the immediate post-irradiation interval without delivery of a second dose. If survival is not dependent upon post-irradiation conditions, one can state that the initial registration of damage produces injury states which are either non-lethal or lethal and the latter cannot be converted to a non-lethal injury state. However, if survival is dependent upon post-irradiation environment, some part of the registered damage may exist in a labile state which may be fixed to a lethal event or repaired permitting survival. If mammalian cells are able to accomplish this kind of repair in the immediate post-irradiation interval, there result important implications for the success of preoperative radiation therapy to reduce the viable tumor cell population to a sufficiently low probability.

Therefore, we next ask the question: Are mammalian cells capable of repairing potentially lethal damage? To study this point, we determined survival of hypoxic tumor cells as a function of time after a single exposure *in vivo*. When such tumors were irradiated with 3000 R, and cells allowed to remain in the hypoxic condition within the irradiated host, survival varied with time (fig. 6). The initial survival increase means that damage, which would have suppressed tumor production, was rapidly repaired.

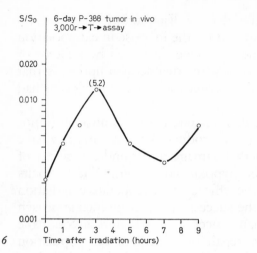
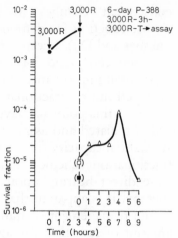

6

7

Fig. 6. Repair of potentially lethal damage by hypoxic (5 day) P-388 tumor cells. Cells were irradiated *in vivo* with 3000 R at time = 0. At times after, cells were removed and assayed for survival.

Fig. 7. Repair of potentially lethal damage by hypoxic (6 day) P-388 tumor cells. Closed circles trace survival increase 3 h after a single dose of 3000 R. Open triangle at time = 0, inner scale, is the survival following a second exposure of 3000 R. The curve traced by the subsequent open triangles traces survival as a function of time after second 3000 R. The closed square is the survival to 6000 R in one exposure; open square, the survival to two doses of 3000 R separated by 3 h as *predicted* from the two dose response of 6-day tumors.

The dip at 9 h and subsequent rise will be discussed below in the context of our results with Chinese hamster cells in culture. These results clearly show that when irradiated hypoxic tumor cells are allowed to remain hypoxic after irradiation, lethal injury is converted to a state which allows cells to divide indefinitely. That the hypoxic state is a necessary requirement for this conversion is seen from the data of similar experiments with one-day (aerobic) tumors. In the latter, survival is not modified by time after a single exposure.

If there is no qualitative difference between sublethal and potentially lethal radiation damage, and if the repair systems for both are the same, one might reasonably expect that the efficiency of potentially lethal damage repair would be influenced by the necessity for the cell to accomplish sublethal damage repair. To test this possibility, animals bearing 6-day tumors were exposed to two doses of 3000 R separated by 3 h. As a function of time after the second dose, cells were assayed for reproductive viability. Figure 7 shows the results of this experiment. The closed circles trace the survival increase three h after 3000 R and gives an estimate of the degree of repair of potentially lethal injury resulting from that exposure. Survival immediately after the second 3000 R is given by the open triangle (zero time after the second 3000 R; total dose = 6000 R). The closed square is the survival expected from an acute exposure of 6000 R; the open square is the survival to two 3000 R exposures separated by 3 h as *predicted* by the 2-dose response of 6-day tumors and demonstrates that the survival to 6000 R delivered in 2 equal fractions separated by 3 h is consistant with our previous results with smaller total doses. The curve traced by the triangles shows survival fluctuations as a function of time in the hypoxic state after the second 3000 R. The points of note are: (1) The initial survival increase is not as rapid as that following a single exposure; (2) substantial survival increase does not occur until 3 h after the second dose; (3) this increase is preceded by an interval during which little or no survival change occurs; (4) the increase in survival is followed by a steep fall. Taken together we conclude that repeated exposures influenced the time-course of potentially lethal damage repair and that the expression of repair by increased survival was delayed as the number of exposures increased.

Therefore, we summarize our findings with mammalian tumor cells *in vivo* as follows: (1) Single-dose response is dependent upon tumor age. Intraperitoneal oxygen tension is a major factor in this regard, although other factors such as nutritional deficiency, changes in age-density-distribution and the presence of a sizable non-growth fraction also play a part. (2) Intraperitoneal hypoxia does not impair the capacity of tumor cells to repair sublethal radiation damage, but hypoxic cells repair such damage less efficiently. (3) When damaged hypoxic cells are provided an aerobic environment, repair proceeds rapidly and efficiently. This finding has obvious implications for our understanding of the radiobiological consequences of reoxygenation during fractionated radiotherapy. (4) If provided a hypoxic post-irradiation environment, tumor cells repair potentially lethal radiation damage. This capacity is modified by prior irradiation and, by implication, the requirement to repair sublethal damage. This suggests that the repair processes for both levels of damage are similar.

2. Chinese Hamster Cells in Culture

The repair of sublethal damage by mammalian cells in culture has been studied extensively [6–13] and the kinetics of repair are well known. We now turn to our evidence that mammalian cells in culture repair potentially lethal damage. Figure 8 shows the results of an experiment in which exponentially growing Chinese hamster cells (V79-103A) were irradiated at time zero and immediately overlayed with Earle's balanced salt solution (EBSS), a bicarbonate buffered solution containing dextrose. At intervals in EBSS at 37°C, sets of dishes were removed, buffer discarded, and cells provided with FS-15 for colony formation. Survival rapidly increased to a maximum after 1 h in EBSS. With longer times in EBSS, survival decreased and was followed by a second rise. The initial increase suggests that mammalian cells in culture repair potentially lethal radiation damage and this observation is similar to that which is typical for liquid holding recovery in bacteria.

It is important to note that the kinetics in figure 8 are similar to those for hypoxic tumor cells *in vivo*. We interpret the dip in survival observed in both cases to mean that during the repair process an unstable molecular state is produced which prevents unlimited division. This is a reasonable suggestion, since part of the repair process may be degradative, and, if interrupted at this point by an environment in which other cell functions (including division) must proceed, radiation damage will be expressed as a lethal event. We interpret the second survival increase to mean that this unstable state exists transiently and is converted to a stable, non-lethal condition with further repair in buffer or in the hypoxic state.

One expectation is that the degradative portion of the repair sequence has a temperature coefficient. To test this assumption we have begun a series of experiments in which cells were incubated in EBSS at 37°C for 2 h after irradiation. Following this interval, warm buffer was replaced by cold buffer and cells incubated at 5°C in a CO_2 controlled environment for intervals up to four hours. Our preliminary results indicate that the dip in survival observed for buffer incubation at 37°C is suppressed by low temperature [5].

Earle's balanced salt solution also provides the required environment for potentially lethal damage repair by P-388 tumor cells. Six-day tumor cells were irradiated *in vivo* and immediately transfered to EBSS at 37°C. As a function of time in buffer, cells were assayed for reproductive viability *in vivo*. Figure 9 shows the results of these experiments. The panel on the left shows the kinetics of repair in buffer at 37°C while that on the right those for incubation at 4°C. In both cases there is rapid increase in survival, although the initial rate and extent of repair at 4°C are depressed. Therefore, hypoxic mammalian tumor cells repair potentially lethal damage *in vivo* or when incubated in EBSS *in vitro*.

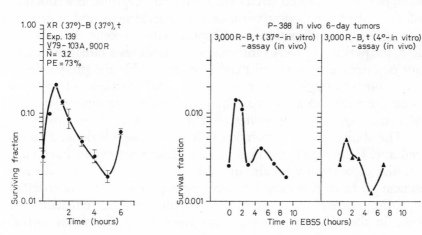

Fig. 8. Survival response of V79-103A Chinese hamster lung cells in culture as a function of time in Earle's balanced salt solution after 900 R. N̄, average number of cells per colony at time = 0; PE, plating efficiency, number of unirradiated cells able to form colonies.
Fig. 9. Repair of potentially lethal damage by P-388 tumor cells in Earle's balanced salt solution (EBSS), *in vitro*, at 37°C or 4°C. Cells were assayed for viability *in vivo*. Cells were irradiated *in vivo* (6-day tumors).

Because survivors to a given radiation dose represent cells which were in resistant response states at the time of exposure, the observed repair kinetics are predominantly for those cells. Thus, the capacity for repairing potentially lethal radiation damage may depend upon cell age. To test this we used synchronous Chinese hamster cells in culture. Prior to harvesting, we incubated monolayers with 2mM hydroxyurea in complete medium for 2 h. Hydroxyurea selectively kills cells which are synthesizing DNA and prevents progression of non-synthesizing cells into the synthetic phase of the cell cycle [14]. Consequently, after a short exposure to this drug, cells accumulate in the pre-synthetic (G_1) phase of the cell cycle. After exposure to hydroxyurea, monolayers were harvested, and resulting single cell suspensions plated.

At intervals after 0.5 h at 37°C (to permit cell attachment) sets of dishes were irradiated with 750 R. Following irradiation at 1 h, 6 h, and 11 h after synchrony, cells were incubated in EBSS for periods up to 6 h. Cells were then refed with FS-15 for colony formation. Figure 10 shows the results of these experiments. In both panels, the closed circles trace survival response as a function of time after synchrony without buffer treatment and represent the age-response-function for Chinese hamster cells. In this cell line, the period of DNA synthesis (S) constitutes a radiation resistant compartment (survival maximum at 4-7 h); the pre-synthetic (G_1), post-synthetic (G_2) and mitotic (M) portions of the cell cycle are radiation sensitive. The open symbols represent survival as a function of time in buffer after irradiation at times shown.

The ability to repair potentially lethal damage is dependent on cell age. Cells which are in middle or late S appear to have substantial capacity for repair, but cells in early or late G_1 do not appear to have this capacity. Because repair of potentially lethal radiation damage is apparently accomplished most efficiently by cells in the process of replicating their DNA, it is not unreasonable to expect that radiation damage repair mechanisms and the replicative process are associated.

WHITMORE and GULYAS [18] have suggested that cells experiencing potentially lethal radiation damage fix that damage to a permanent lethal event relatively rapidly after irradiation. From the results of ELKIND, HAN and VOLZ [7] we know that cells not destined to form macroscopic colonies are able to accomplish one or two post-irradiation divisions before reproductive death occurs. Because the only necessary and sufficient condition for the production of a colony is that at least one cell be viable, a microcolony may contain cells which are nonviable. Therefore, although the damage initially registered in the parent cell may not have been sufficient to suppress eventual colony formation, one or more of the progeny resulting from the first, second or third post-irradiation division may, nonetheless, be nonviable. A question of importance, therefore, is whether lethal damage segregated into daughter or granddaughter cells is repairable. We have designed experiments which provide insight into this question.

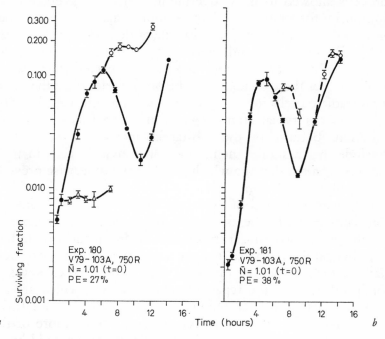

Fig. 10 a and *b*. Two experiments showing survival to 750 R as a function of time after synchronization with 2.0 mm hydroxyurea, 2 h. Closed circles show survival without buffer treatment after irradiation. Open symbols trace survival as a function of time in buffer after exposure at times indicated by appropriate closed circle. Low plating efficiencies reflect cell killing by hydroxyurea in original population. Courtesy of Belli and Shelton [4].

If daughter cells are not able to repair segregated lethal damage, survival fluctuations should not be observed when incubation in EBSS is delayed until the post-irradiation multiplicity reaches 2-3. On the other hand, if such damage is repairable, survival increase, at least for short incubation times in buffer, should be observed. We have done two kinds of experiments. First, incubation of microcolonies in buffer for intervals has been followed by trypsinization to allow single cells to express colony formation. The second kind of experiment was designed to answer the question: Does the association of nonviable and viable cells in a microcolony affect the repair process?

In figure 11, are shown the results of an experiment in which single cells were irradiated, refed with complete growth medium and cells allowed to grow overnight. When the average colony multiplicity for irradiated cells was approximately 3 (zero time in figure 11), growth medium was discarded and replaced with EBSS. The open diamonds trace the growth of irradiated cells in buffer at 37°C over a period of 3 h. As expected, there was no growth under these conditions. The open circles trace the growth of unirradiated cells in medium over the same interval. The closed circles trace survival after intervals in EBSS followed by trypsinization. Because of the substantial increase in survival, we conclude that a significant number of nonviable cells in microcolonies repaired damage which would have otherwise prevented their unlimited division.

However, this kind of experiment does not provide information with regard to the association of viable and nonviable cells within the microcolony. If trypsinization after incubation in buffer is omitted, and no survival increase is observed, it can be concluded that the survival increase observed with trypsinized cells was predominantly due to the repair of nonviable cells which are associated with viable cells in the microcolony. However, if all of the cells in a microcolony are nonviable, and one or more of them repair potentially lethal damage, survival increase should be seen with incubation in buffer because eventual colony formation requires only one viable cell. In figure 12, survival fraction is plotted as a function of time in EBSS at a time when the average colony multiplicity after irradiation was 2.1. The open triangle is the survival to 800 R, without buffer, but after trypsinization of microcolonies. The results clearly show that a substantial fraction of the repaired population is derived from cells which were contained in colonies in which all of the members were nonviable. In order to observe the kind of result seen in figure 12, at least one of the cells in a nonviable microcolony must repair damage.

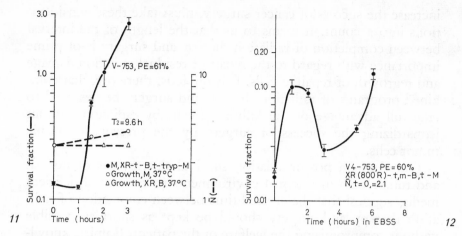

Fig. 11. Repair of potentially lethal damage by daughter cells. V-753 Chinese hamster cells in culture. Open triangles show growth of irradiated cells incubated in buffer at 37°C; open circles, growth of unirradiated cells in complete medium at 37°C. Closed circles trace the survival of irradiated cells allowed to grow to a multiplicity ($\overline{\mathrm{N}}$) of 2.8 and incubated in buffer for various intervals followed by colony dispersion with trypsin (0.05%). Times are times in buffer (closed circles and open triangles) or medium (open circles).

Fig. 12. Survival of microcolonies arising from irradiated cells as a function of time in buffer. $\overline{\mathrm{N}}$ at time = 0, 2.1. The open triangle gives the survival for cells from trypsinized colonies not incubated in buffer.

Therefore, the association of viable and nonviable cells within a microcolony does not influence the repair process. In addition, the similarity between the kinetics here and those seen with cells incubated in EBSS immediately after irradiation (parent cells, fig. 5) suggests that the repair process is the same in daughter and parent cells and that the cellular systems responsible for repairing potentially lethal radiation damage are transferred from parent to progeny unchanged and are not affected by the presence of radiation damage.

Summary and Conclusions

We have shown that mammalian cells of normal and malignant origin are capable of repairing sublethal and potentially lethal radiation damage under a variety of environmental conditions. Any preoperative radiotherapeutic scheme which is designed to increase the success of cancer surgery, must take these considerations into account. It seems to us that the length of the interval between completion of radiation therapy and surgery is of prime importance with regard to the repair of residual radiation damage and regrowth of repaired cells. It is obvious, therefore, that combined programs of radiation therapy and surgery be designed to take full advantage of the killing of cells by radiation without jeopardizing the success of surgery by the presence of viable tumor cells.

Our data on post-irradiation survival fluctuations of normal and tumor cells in minimal environments (hypoxia and deficient media) suggest that the elapsed time between completion of radiation therapy and surgery should be kept as short as possible without compromising the welfare of the patient. Empiric knowledge and clinical experience are valuable in predicting the degree of restitution of surgically stressed, irradiated normal tissues. On the other hand, radiation damage repair by tumor cells in the interval between completion of radiation therapy will, in large part, determine size of the viable tumor cell population at the time of surgery. As our understanding of the cellular processes occurring after irradiation increases, in particular, of those processes responsible for damage repair in parent and daughter cells as influenced by such factors as reoxygenation and cell division, we will derive a more rational approach to combined radiotherapeutic and surgical management of human cancer.

References

1. BELLI, J. A. and ANDREWS, J. R.: Relationship between tumor growth and radiosensitivity. J. nat. Cancer Inst. 31: 689–703 (1963).
2. BELLI, J. A.; DICUS, G. J. and BONTE, F. J.: Radiation response of mammalian tumor cells. I. Repair of sublethal damage in vivo. J. nat. Cancer Inst. 38: 673–682 (1967).
3. BELLI, J. A. and ROACH, A.: Anoxic radiation response in cultured mammalian cells. Brit. J. Radiol. 41: 390–391 (1968).
4. BELLI, J. A. and SHELTON, M.: Potentially lethal radiation damage: Repair by mammalian cells in culture. Science 165: 490–492 (1969).
5. BELLI, J. A. Unpublished results.
6. ELKIND, M. M. and SUTTON, H.: Radiation response of mammalian cells grown in culture. I. Repair of X-ray damage in surviving Chinese hamster cells. Radiat. Res. 13: 556–593 (1960).

7. ELKIND, M. M.; HAN, A. and VOLZ, K. W.: Radiation response of mammalian cells grown in culture. IV. Dose dependence of division delay and post-irradiation growth of surviving and non-surviving Chinese hamster cells. J. nat. Cancer Inst. *30:* 705–725 (1963).

8. ELKIND, M. M.; SUTTON-GILBERT, H.; MOSES, W. B.; ALESCIO, T. and SWAIN, R. W.: Radiation response of mammalian cells grown in culture. V. Temperature dependence of the repair of X-ray damage in surviving cells (aerobic and hypoxic). Radiat. Res. *25:* 359–376 (1965).

9. ELKIND, M. M.; WITHERS, H. R. and BELLI, J. A.: Intracellular repair and the oxygen effect in radiobiology and radiotherapy; Front. Rad. Ther. Onc., vol. *3*, pp. 55–87 (1968).

10. HEWITT, H. B.: Studies of the dissemination and quantitative transplantation of a lymphocytic leukaemia of CBA mice. Brit. J. Cancer *12:* 378–401 (1958).

11. HEWITT, H. B. and WILSON, C. W.: A survival curve for mammalian leukaemia cells irradiated *in vivo* (implications for the treatment of mouse leukaemia by whole-body irradiation). Brit. J. Cancer *13:* 69–75 (1959).

12. PUCK, T. T. and MARCUS, P. I.: A rapid method for viable cell titration and clone production with HeLa cells in tissue culture: The use of X-irradiated cells to supply conditioning factors. Proc. nat. Acad. Sci., Wash. *41:* 432–437 (1955).

13. SINCLAIR, W. K. and MORTON, R. A.: Recovery following X-irradiation of synchronized Chinese hamster cells. Nature, Lond. *203:* 247–250 (1964).

14. SINCLAIR, W. K. and MORTON, R. A.: X-ray sensitivity during the cell generation cycle of cultured Chinese hamster cells. Radiat. Res. *29:* 450–474 (1966).

15. SUIT, H. D. and MAEDA, M. M.: Hyperbaric oxygen and the radiobiology of a C3H mouse mammary carcinoma. J. nat. Cancer Inst. *39:* 639–652 (1967).

16. THOMLINSON, R. H.: The effect of fractionated irradiation on the proportion of anoxic cells in an intact experimental tumor. Brit. J. Radiol. *39:* 158 (1966).

17. VAN PUTTEN, L. M. and KALLMAN, R. F.: Oxygenation states of a transplantable tumor during fractionated radiation therapy. J. nat. Cancer Inst. *40:* 441–451 (1968).

18. WHITMORE, G. F. and GULYAS, S.: Studies on recovery processes in mouse L cells. Nat. Cancer Inst. Monogr. *24:* 141–156 (1967).

Authors' addresses: Dr. J. A. BELLI, Department of Radiotherapy, Harvard Medical School, *Boston, MA;* Miss G. J. DICUS, Biology Division, The University of Texas at Dallas, *Dallas, TX;* Mr. W. NAGLE, Department of Radiology, The University of Texas Southwestern Medical School at Dallas, *Dallas, TX* (USA).

Front. Radiation Ther. Onc., vol. 5, pp. 58–71
(Karger, Basel/München/Paris/New York 1970)

Investigative Aspects of Preoperative Irradiation for Advanced Carcinoma of the Larynx and Laryngopharynx

J. L. GOLDMAN and W. H. FRIEDMAN

Department of Otolaryngology (Director: Prof. J. L. GOLDMAN), Mount Sinai Hospital and
City Hospital Center, Queens, New York, N. Y.

Radiation therapy and surgery have long been separate, successful modalities for treating small and intrinsic carcinomas of the larynx. Since Coutard introduced the modern, protracted, fractional method of irradiation in the 1920's, the 5-year survival rate of patients with intrinsic vocal cord lesions has been over 80% using either modality. However, prior to 1958, advanced carcinomas of the larynx and laryngopharynx presented a problem which neither modality solved with significant success. The cure rate for extrinsic lesions, particularly posterolateral, supraglottic cancers was approximately twenty percent. Only one of five patients with this disease lived 5 years after treatment with radiation alone or surgery alone! Various combinations of surgery and radiation had been tried with indifferent results, notably the 'sandwich' technique of pre- and postoperative radiation, and the most common combination, salvage surgery for radiation failures or palliative radiation for surgical failures. Confronted with this problem, a concept of combined preoperative radiation and radical surgery for advanced carcinoma of the larynx and laryngopharynx was introduced in the Department of Otolaryngology of The Mount Sinai Hospital in 1958. This plan was conceived as an uncompromising program of high dosage irradiation administered in fractions over a six-week period followed by a three to five week interval waiting period, followed by laryngectomy, ipsilateral hemithyroidectomy, and radical neck dissection regardless of the tumor response to irradiation. All patients included in this program were those classified as Stage III as determined by the VIIth

International Congress of Cancer, patients with lesions involving more than one anatomic region of the larynx or laryngopharynx with or without unilateral or bilateral cervical metastases.

In a sense, the entire Combined Therapy Program was an investigative effort, since this was the first program of its kind. We had no precedent, and in establishing a protocol it was necessary, at times, to be arbitrary. The dosage of 5,500 rads of Cobalt 60 teletherapy was selected partly because radiation physiologists had established a sigmoid curve demonstrating the lethal effect of irradiation on cancer cells at that level, but principally because previous experience had indicated that this was the maximum dosage of radiotherapy consistent with safe, effective surgery. The interval waiting period of 3 to 5 weeks was based on the average time required for the initial radiation reaction to subside. The surgery, wide field laryngectomy, ipsilateral radical neck dissection and hemithyroidectomy, is always based on pre-radiation maps of the lesion for reasons which I will explain.

Since 1958, 53 patients have been treated with Combined Therapy. Thirty-five are alive and well. Six are dead of disease and twelve patients died of other causes. Using the International Classification, the 5-year survival rate for Stage III is 86% deter-

Table I. Survival rates

		International classification					
		5-Year		3-Year		2-Year	
Stage III	Determinate	18/21	86%	33/36	92%	44/46	96%
	Absolute	18/27	67%	33/40	83%	44/49	90%
		American classification					
		5-Year		3-Year		2-Year	
Stage II	Determinate	2/2	100%	10/10	100%	17/17	100%
	Absolute	2/5	40%	10/11	91%	17/17	100%
Stage III	Determinate	4/5	80%	8/9	89%	9/9	100%
	Absolute	4/7	57%	8/10	80%	9/10	90%
Stage IV	Determinate	12/14	86%	15/17	88%	18/20	90%
	Absolute	12/15	80%	15/19	79%	18/22	82%

minate and 67% absolute (table I). The 3-year survival rate is 92% determinate and 83% absolute. Using the classification of the American Joint Committee on Cancer Staging and End Results Reporting, the 5-year survival rate for Stage II is 100% determinate and 40% absolute; for Stage III 80% determinate and 57% absolute; and for Stage IV 86% determinate and 91% absolute. The three year survival rate for Stage II is 100% determinate and 91% absolute; for Stage III 89% determinate and 80% absolute; and for Stage IV 88% determinate and 79% absolute.

Because of the initial clinical effectiveness of the Combined Therapy Program, a histopathological study of resected laryngeal and neck specimens was begun in 1961 to determine precisely the effects of radiotherapy on laryngeal cancer. Surgical specimens consisting of larynx or laryngopharynx, neck specimens, and ipsilateral hemithyroid gland were taken directly from the operating room to our laboratory. The larynx and extrinsic muscles were dissected free from the neck specimen and placed in 20% formalin. The sternocleidomastoid muscle was dissected from the remaining neck specimen and sent to the pathology laboratory for routine study. Neck tissue was affixed to cork board so that its configuration resembled the natural anatomic configuration in the neck. This tissue was then immersed in 10% formalin.

The technique for preparing laryngeal and neck specimens for histologic study has been described in a previous publication. The specimens are embedded in celloidin and serial, en bloc sections are obtained of the entire larynx and neck specimens. Every tenth section is stained with hematoxylin and eosin, and if negative for tumor, every fifth section is stained. In this way, the chances of missing a microscopic focus of laryngeal cancer are remote. Every lymph node is automatically included in the pathological examination of the neck. To date, 18 larynges and 15 neck specimens have been studied in this fashion.

Larynges

The response of laryngeal cancer to radiotherapy included a wide spectrum of radiation induced fibrosis. Inflammatory cells were elicited with a characteristic giant cell response (fig. 1) and eventual invasion by fibroblasts. Mature fibrous tissue resulted which surrounded and replaced tumor remnants (fig. 2). Endothelial proliferation and fibrous obliteration of the lumens of small arteries was a related response which probably resulted in hypoxia.

Laryngeal tumors most often responded to radiotherapy by regression to isolated islands of cells in a random distribution throughout the original tumor site. These islands existed under intact mucous membrane (fig. 3). They regressed to areas not accessible by biopsy (fig. 4) and we have seen cancer cells as far as 1.5 cm from the mucosal surface from which they presumably originated (fig. 5). These findings suggested that laryngeal neoplasms do not respond to radiotherapy by centripetal regression, and that the entire tumor site observed prior to radiation must be excised. Examination of the patient's larynx either indirectly or directly following radiotherapy might fail to reveal the presence of a submucosal nest of cells lurking well below an apparently 'cured' mucous membrane. Our serial section studies revealed that 10 out of 13 clinically negative contained microscopic cancer. For this reason, preradiation maps of the original lesion are vital; and, unfortunately, the post-radiation appearance of a larynx completely devoid of clinical evidence of cancer is deceiving and dangerous to the patient if there is a resultant decision not to operate.

Neck Specimens

Serial sections of radical neck dissection specimens revealed surprising clinical as well as histologic information. Of 11 patients who had palpable nodes prior to radiation therapy, seven were completely free of tumor on serial section examination of the neck specimens. Of four elective neck dissections, one contained a normal sized lymph node with microscopic evidence of cancer.

In 53 cases there has been no ipsilateral cervical recurrence and only two cases of contralateral recurrence, both of which occurred in patients with anaplastic cancer. There were three other local recurrences, in the ipsilateral thyroid, tongue and esophagostome.

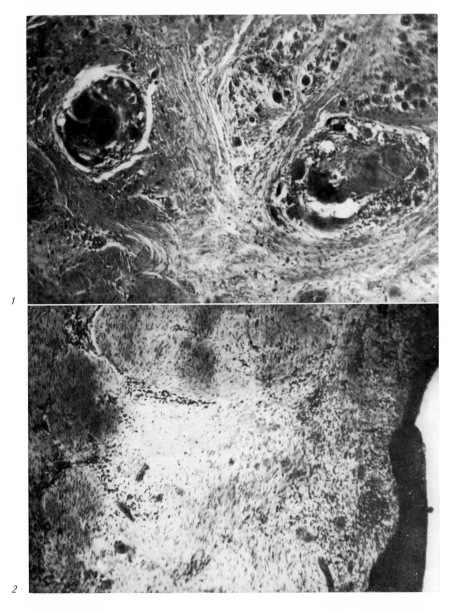

Fig. 1. Foreign body giant cells containing fully keratinized pearls in region formerly occupied by cancer.

Fig. 2. Fibrous tissue replacing area formerly occupied by cancer.

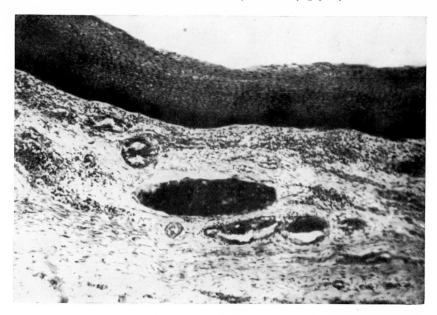

Fig. 3. Cancer focus beneath an intact laryngeal mucosa.

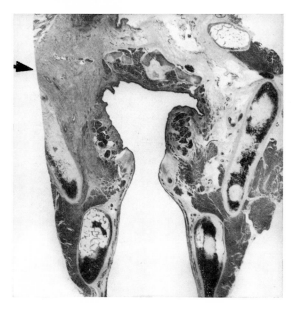

Fig. 4. Tiny focus of cancer approximately 1.5 cm from intact mucous membrane.

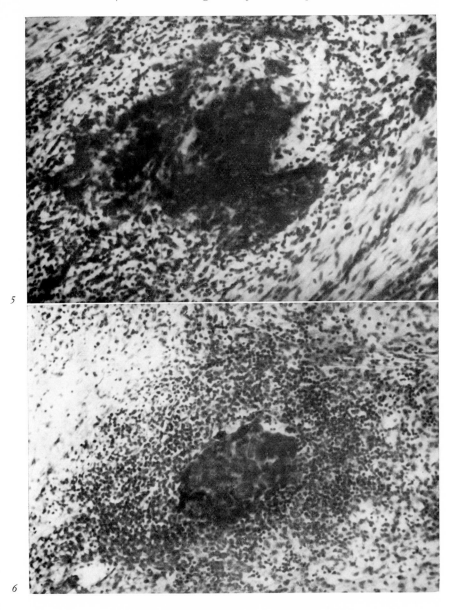

5

6

Fig. 5. High power view of cancer nest shown in previous illustration.
Fig. 6. Focus of cancer in a cervical lymph node following radiotherapy. Inflammatory cells are seen infiltrating the capsule and surrounding the neoplasm.

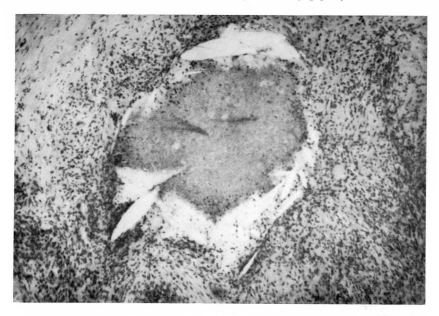

Fig. 7. Total replacement of cervical lymph node with fibrous tissue.

Following irradiation, cervical lymph nodes shrank in size. Fixed nodes became mobile and small mobile nodes often disappeared clinically. Serial sections revealed that cancer was often completely destroyed by radiation and residual cancer was surrounded by fibrous tissue. No evidence of a cancer focus outside a lymph node was noted.

A variety of other radiations reactions were demonstrated, including infiltration of the capsules of lymph nodes with inflammatory cells (fig. 6) and progression to encapsulation (fig. 7) or replacement of tumor with fibrous tissue.

Cell Viability

The question of cell viability has often intrigued the laryngologist and radiotherapist who, as we have seen, have no absolute parameters for measuring the effectiveness of radiotherapy on advanced cancer of the larynx. Since the effects of radiotherapy are determined by ionizing events within the laryngeal cancer cells, it seemed logical that we should make some attempt at following the progress of radiotherapy at cellular and radiobiologic levels, hopefully to determine the killing effect of radiation and the viability of residual cancer cells. To facilitate this we have monitored the effects of preoperative radiation on the death and recovery of laryngeal cancer cells using tritiated thymidine autoradiography. Cell viability can be established unequivocally by the presence of intranuclear tritium and, more important, predictions of the behavior of tumors can be based on biologic as well as histologic criteria.

Four patients with cancer of the larynx have been studied in this fashion. The technique utilized, as demonstrated by JOHNSON and BOND in their 1961 study of human breast tumors, appears in a previous publication [7]. Biopsy specimens of laryngeal cancer were taken prior to radiotherapy and during the course of irradiation. At the completion of surgery, the entire tumor bearing area of the larynx was removed and sectioned. These specimens of living tissue were incubated with tritiated thymidine for 30 minutes in tissue culture media. Following incubation radioautograms were prepared.

The 30-minute *in vitro* exposure time included only a small fraction of the cell cycle. Thymidine was incorporated exclusively into DNA during the eight hour 'S' or synthesis phase of the cycle. Therefore, only those cells in the 'S' phase, or those cells actually synthesizing DNA, incorporated thymidine and became tagged with the attached tritium (fig. 8). In each patient a laryngeal biopsy was taken for autoradiography following pathologic diagnosis of the lesion prior to radiotherapy. Heavy labelling was seen in each of these non-radiated squamous cell cancer biopsy specimens (fig. 9). As many as ten cells per high power field were labelled, with grain counts ranging from 10 to 30 grains per labelled cell. Following 3,500 rads of Cobalt 60 teletherapy, there was in each case a marked reduction in both the number of labelled cells per high power field, and in the number of grains per labelled nucleus. Slide after slide of necrotic, non-labelled tumor was seen at the 3,500 rads level with only islands of viable tumor remaining (fig. 10). In addition, we saw routine histologic confirmation of tumor necrosis with pyknotic nuclei, vacuolated cytoplasm, and cellular debris.

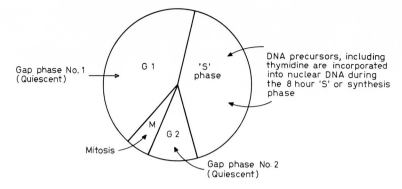

Fig. 8. The mammalian cell cycle and relative areas representing phase sequence.

At surgery, the previously biopsied tumor bearing areas were removed from the laryngectomy specimens and incubated with tritiated thymidine as previously described. This, in each case, followed the prescribed 5,500 rads course of preoperative irradiation and the three to six week interval waiting period. All four patients demonstrated a similar picture. Characteristically, labelling occurred in widely separated tiny foci measuring approximately 500 μm to 1,000 μm in diameter. Surprisingly, labelling in these areas was abundant (fig. 11). As many as 10 to 12 labelled cells per high power field were found. No cell, however, exposed more than 12 grains. In addition, very little histologic evidence of radiation damage appeared in these labelled foci.

Autoradiography, then, with tritiated thymidine has shown repetitive diminution of cell labelling with the progress of radiotherapy. Unequivocally viable areas have been demonstrated in tumors which had clinically disappeared. This was predictable, since tumors often recur following dosages of radiotherapy much greater than 5,500 rads.

The isolated but exuberant labelling seen in our patients following 5,500 rads may have represented partial synchronization by irradiation. In each case, the maximum number of labelled cells per high power field exceeded the number seen at 3,500 rads, but the grain count was always less than the non-irradiated

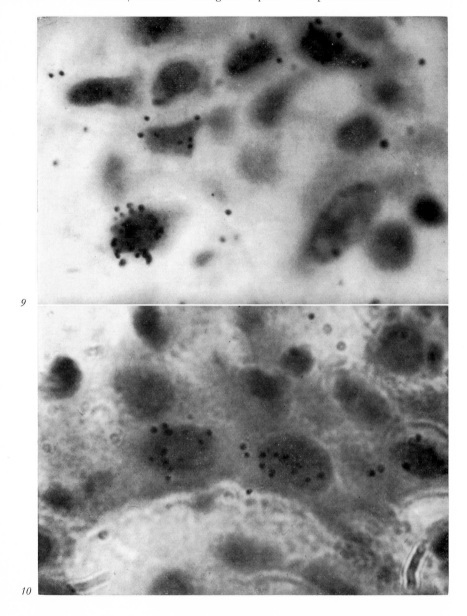

Fig. 9. Biopsy of squamous cell carcinoma of the larynx incubated with tritiated thymidine prior to irradiation.
Fig. 10. Less labelling per unit field and less label density per cell are seen in this biopsy specimen taken following 3,500 rads Cobalt 60 preoperative irradiation.

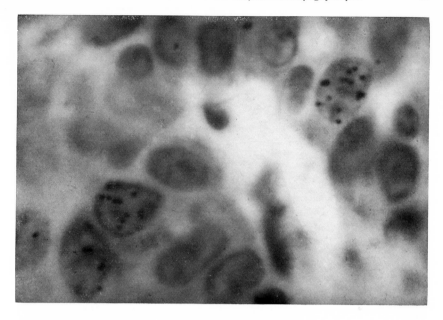

Fig. 11. Surgical specimen removed after 5,500 rads Cobalt 60 ands a 5-week waiting period. Note abundant labelling and absence of tissue reaction.

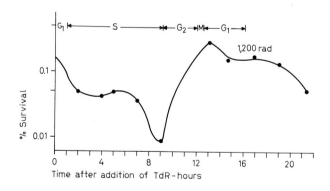

Fig. 12. Survival curve of a partially synchronized population of 'L' cells in tissue culture suspension following a single exposure of 1,200 rads. Note extreme radiosensitivity of late 'S' phase. (From GULYAS and BOTOND: Radiation sensitivity throughout the cell cycle and its relation to recovery; Cellular Radiation Biology, p. 423; Williams & Wilkins, Baltimore 1964.)

specimens. It appeared that many cells surviving irradiation were in the same phase – or synchronous – and therefore appeared labelled at the same time. It can be assumed that if these cells could be monitored so that we know exactly when the majority are in the 'S' phase, a better effect might be expected from radiotherapy applied at that time. It has been shown that tumors in the 'S' phase of the cell cycle are more radiosensitive than at other times. GULYAS and BOTOND [6] demonstrated a tenfold increase in radio-sensitivity during the 'S' phase utilizing a suspension of L cells partially synchronized by previous irradiation (fig. 12). In the future, chemotherapeutic agents such as dactinomycin and colchicine may be utilized in conjunction with radiotherapy so that partial or complete synchronization can be achieved.

Summary

(1) The Combined Therapy Program for treatment of advanced cancer of the larynx and laryngopharynx is presented as an investigative effort which has become a matter of clinical routine because of the apparent increase in patient survival. (2) Reasons for this increase have been partially elaborated in the histopathology laboratory where it has been shown that large laryngeal tumors often regress to isolated, random foci of submucosal tumor islands. This has supported our contention that the original tumor bearing area must be removed regardless of the response to radiotherapy. (3) En bloc serial section studies of neck dissection specimens have revealed a spectrum of radiation induced fibrous replacement of tumor bearing lymph nodes, probably altering the progress of cervical metastatic disease. (4) Tritiated thymidine studies of radiated laryngeal cancer has shown repetitive diminution of cell labelling with the progress of radiotherapy with exuberant labelling in isolated foci still present at the time of laryngectomy.

References

1. GOLDMAN, J. L., and SILVERSTONE, S. M.: Combined radiation and surgical therapy for cancer of the larynx and laryngopharynx. Trans. amer. Acad. Ophthalmol. Otolaryngol. 65: 496–507 (1961).
2. GOLDMAN, J. L.; SILVERSTONE, S. M.; ROSIN, H. D.; CHEREN, R. V., and ZAK, F. G.: Combined radiation and surgical therapy for cancer of the larynx and laryngopharynx II. Laryngoscope 74: 1,111–1,134 (1964).
3. GOLDMAN, J. L.; CHEREN, R. V.; ZAK, F. G., and GUNSBERG, M. J.: Histopathology of larynges and radical neck specimens. Ann. Otol. 75: 1–23 (1966).
4. GOLDMAN, J. L. and FRIEDMAN, W. H.: The intranuclear tracer, cell viability, and pre-operative irradiation. Laryngoscope 72: 1,315–1,327 (1967).
5. GOLDMAN, J. L.; BLOOM, B. S.; ZAK, F. G.; FRIEDMAN, W. H.; GUNSBERG, M. J., and SILVERSTONE, S. M.: Serial microscopic studies of radical neck dissections. Arch. Otol. 89: 620–628 (1969).

6. GULYAS, S. and BOTOND, J.: Radiation sensitivity throughout the cell cycle and its relationship to recovery ; in WHITMORE Cellular radiation biology (Williams & Wilkins, Baltimore 1965).

7. JOHNSON, H. A. and BOND, V. P.: Method of labelling tissues with tritiated thymidine *in vitro* and its use in comparing rates of cell proliferation in duct epithelium, fibroadenoma, and carcinoma of human breast. Cancer *14:* 639–643 (1961).

8. LEROUX-ROBERT, J.: Etude statistique de 644 cas de cancers du larynx et de l'hypopharynx traités par chirurgie aux associations radio-chirurgicales. Ann. oto-rhino-laryng., Paris *76:* 533–566 (1959).

9. NABRE, M. O. R.: Clinical stage classification of malignant tumors of the larynx. Acta Un. int. Cancer *16:* 1,865–1,873 (1960).

10. SILVERSTONE, S. M.; GOLDMAN, J. L., and ROSIN, H. D.: Combined therapy irradiation and surgery, for advanced cancer of the laryngopharynx. Amer. J. of Roentgenol. *90:* 1,023–1,031 (1963).

11. SMITH, R. R.; CAULK, R. M.; RUSSELL, W. O., and JACKSON, C. L.: End results in 600 laryngeal cancers using the American Joint Committee's proposed method of stage classification and end results reporting. Surg. Gynec. Obstet. *113:* 435–444 (1961).

Authors' address: Dr. J. L. GOLDMAN and Dr. W. H. FRIEDMAN, Department of Otolaryngology, Mount Sinai Hospital and City Hospital Center, Queens, *New York, NY* (USA).

Front. Radiation Ther. Onc., vol. 5, pp. 72–92
(Karger, Basel/München/Paris/New York 1970)

What can we Believe? Some Observations
on the Design of Clinical Investigations

I. D. ROTKIN

Associate Professor of Preventive Medicine and Community Health, University of Illinois
at the Medical Center, Chicago, Ill.; and Lecturer in Epidemiology and Community Health,
School of Medicine, University of California, San Diego, Calif.

The key to the control of clinical trials is randomization. You hypothesize that one treatment is superior to another, and you test this belief with a plan so controlled by randomization that bias and error are minimized. Yet, despite inferential pitfalls traditionally described as one kind of error or another, randomization may not always be the perfect statistical leveller we think it is.

It has become commonplace to refer to disastrous consequences of experimental inference as 'errors' of the first and second kind. In terms of therapy, these are the statistical statements that one treatment appears more effective than another but is not, an error of the first kind; or that both treatments are not substantially different in effect when one really is appreciably better, an error of the second kind. Since these unfortunate consequences of trials may result from combinations of error and the interference of unknown influences, perhaps they could more aptly be regarded as empirical hazards or false conclusions.

As many know, results from therapeutic trials most often are far from spectacular, and differences of effect between two competing treatments seldom are of a convincing percentage magnitude. Where there is a sweeping miraculous change, trials may not even be needed because where previously nobody survived after onset of an inexorable disease process, or survival was uniformly short, now perhaps everyone survives and pathology disappears. Except for annoying doubts about longterm side effects it is an improvement to survive, and trials are not required. But this dramatic degree of cure potential seldom happens in medical history, and the problem generally is to make quite sure that the new treatment is superior without additional risk to the patient. Since this is difficult to do, fanatical adherence to the experimental design is important, and randomization plus adequately large sample sizes promote some measure of protection against errors of the various kinds, and also lend some credibility to results.

But this assumes that your project truly is controlled. With humans this is to say that *all* influences bearing upon the endpoint, whether survival, tumor regression, palliation or restoration to usefulness, are evenly and equally distributed in both groups of patients you are comparing. The fact that you have controlled a few known variables by randomization does not necessarily mean you have maximally controlled all influences, because events in life tend sometimes to hang together in linkages. Given a universe of variables, some will distribute differently from others, not only by chance, but by preferential interaction with others. This is not as true with animal experiments, and I will briefly compare animal work with human programs later in this talk. Some of you are more expert than I in the area of trials, but I am told that others have not been exposed to this kind of reasoning. There will be no statistics or formulas because technicalities are available in full detail from textbooks and the general literature.

Objectives of a Controlled Clinical Program

We are here interested in cancer as a disease process, and specifically in the treatment and control of cancer. The questions are simple and always the same:

1. Given two competing treatments for the same site-specific tumor, which is more effective?
2. Is it really convincingly superior?
3. How much advantage does it confer?
4. Does it carry hazards which rule it out?
5. What value or measure or endpoint are we willing to accept in appraising the superiority of such a treatment?
6. What influences might interefere with a correct appraisal, and can they be neutralized, understood, and adjusted?

The need for a clinical trial arises when through speculation, accidental discovery, or laboratory experiments with animals, the possibility of an improved treatment is uncovered, whether by radiotherapy or surgery or chemotherapy, or by any combination of these; or when in retrospect the individual responses of patients to a change in procedure seem to endorse a followup investigation. The hypothesis always is that the new treatment is advantageous over the accepted treatment of choice. A design now must be contrived to test this hypothesis.

Trial Structure

Two avenues are open: a search for anecdotal material, or a controlled clinical trial. Anecdotal material requires the collection of case histories describing differential responses of patients to previous treatments, and perhaps improvement from modifications.

The evaluation of chart material carries inherent difficulties:

1. Where a treatment was modified, exposure to the first treatment may have been eventful, but the effect was delayed and wrongly ascribed to the new course.
2. Even when case histories are used retrospectively as controls in comparing with patients currently under modified treatment, such a comparison is doubtfully valid because control patients were treated at different times and under different conditions.
3. The auditing of medical records as they are now maintained seldom is a satisfactory procedure.
4. Individual efforts and reports by different physicians are not dependably uniform, and there is no way in which to evaluate such data.

However, collected case material may be useful in searching for variables which can distinguish responders from nonresponders. Such a study was reported by Keller et al. [6], where histologic classification of Hodgkin's Disease was applied retrospectively to evaluate a series of untreated cases. Several pathologists independently assigned these cases to separate histologic classes, with a fairly high degree of rating correlation. From these results, an index was proposed which combined histologic and staging data for prediction of five year survival, and with which patients could be partitioned into those groups which respond more or less favorably to radiotherapy. Studies of this type can be valuable in establishing variables for the design of trials, especially where collected pathologic specimens are available for review.

Control Studies

In theory, a control study or trial has two major aspects:

1. All possible variables which may conspire to obscure evaluation of competing treatments are controlled. This leaves only the criterion variable, the treatment, for appraisal.
2. One group of patients, treated with one modality, is compared against another *similar* group, treated with the other.

In practice, both objectives are met by sampling patients who are described by a set of variables such as age, size and histology of tumor, and perhaps several others. All remaining possibly associated factors reputedly are controlled by randomization, so the total of patient of one group is exactly like the total of patients in the other group. It stands to reason that if one group responds more effectively to one treatment than the other group, a superior modality has been demonstrated. This is like applying one treatment to a group of patients, then somehow wiping out the treatment as if it had never existed and applying the second to the same group.

Endpoints

In evaluating the advantage of one therapeutic procedure over another, an agreement is required on some reasonable measure of improvement. One of the debated issues of clinical trials is whether survival rates are an adequate dimension for estimates of treatment effectiveness. There are others: tumor regression, and recurrence rates and patterns. LARIONOV [7] lists these endpoints as: (1) Changes in the tumor involving arrest of growth, and partial and compete regression. (2) Changes in the body, including recovery of work capacity. (3) Time parameters, including the beginning of therapeutic effect, time of maximum effect, and duration of the effect before relapse, and (4) reproducibility of the therapeutic effect.

His emphasis on the recovery of work capacity, with indicators such as mobility and a sense of wellbeing, is reflected by the current

medical interest in the whole person and in the meaningfulness of continued existence, but there are difficulties in measuring the patient's
return to usefulness with any degree of reproducible precision. In
discussing survivals as an objective endpoint, CORNFIELD [3] suggests that other endpoints are possible, such as the ability to swallow in
esophageal cancer, a demonstrable response criterion. However, this
in itself can be subjective.

Sampling, Bias, Error

If you don't already know this, you will learn that as the size of
your experimental groups increase, smaller significant differences
between them can be found, and you can actualize what you can
believe with greater precision. Your statistician will tell you
to begin your trials by first estimating the number of cases you will
need to attain a reasonable level of credibility. There are tables,
FISHER's [5] and others, which tell you how many patients to
include in each of your two comparison groups so that your
chance of failing to detect a significant difference between both
groups bears no more than a certain likelihood. If you are satisfied
with larger differences you can get along with fewer cases, but if
you have fewer cases you may lose smaller but important differences which exist. If you want to detect very small meaningful differences in survival rates or other endpoints, you will need staggeringly
large numbers of cases. This is the reason for cooperatively extending clinical trials to several participating institutions.

  Sources of bias usually are (1) lack of comparability of one trial
group with the other, (2) derivation of patients from different
institutions than controls, (3) comparison of patients obtained at one
time with controls sampled another time, (4) differences in tumor
histopathology, (5) failure to conform to the design of the program.

Randomization

Simple randomization consists of drawing each patient by chance
from the pool of all possible and available patients with the
same lesion, and assigning him to one of two competing groups,
A and B. Tables of random numbers often are used for this,

although other devices may be suitable. If large numbers of patients are available and the population is homogeneous, simple random selection may be adequate, but more often sample sizes are limited. From reference animal work or retrospective human experience, it may be possible to anticipate some of the factors influencing prognosis, and to stratify each sample according to these. Stratified randomization is the method most often used in comparing populations, including political surveys. You can't compare young with old, rich with poor, educated with illiterate. Similarly, with diseased groups it is best to divide each sample according to some plan, stratifying for site of the lesion, pathology, age and sex, and other factors which must be held constant. This results in similar subgroups for each major trial group. The possibility of using a matched-pair design exists, where one patient is matched against another for such a group of variables, and each member of the pair receives alternate treatments. This can be effective and is used in behavioral and risk factor studies. It results in rigid control, but is very difficult to achieve within limited time for more than perhaps three variables, because the pool of patients must be very large in order to discover pairs of perfectly matching individuals. It is much easier in risk factor studies, where you compare a diseased person with one who does not have that disease. However, such a design may lend itself to nonparametric statistical tests which are economical and direct.

There are many published examples of randomized designs, and some good generalized discussion of cooperative clinical programs with collaborative protocols. DEELEY [4] is a resource for an understanding not only of randomized designs, but also of controlled clinical trials. CORNFIELD [3] has contributed valuable remarks on the structure of a cooperative experiment. His material applies directly to radiotherapy, as does also WATSON's [10], who has summarized what the others have said, and who provides guidelines for clinical trials in a radiotherapy center.

Meaningfulness of Results

Survival for a set length of time is the most often used endpoint, but as SCHNEIDERMAN [9], LARIONOV [7], and others have pointed out, this can include just barely keeping a patient alive. Regression of the tumor might be considered more convenient because finalized data must be postponed until survival runs out for all patients, but measurement of the tumor is not necessarily an indication that recurrence will not take place, and perhaps soon; or that the patient will be able to return to useful life. Also, one must be convinced that regression is associated with survival.

What may be most important is that some patients may respond more readily because they are endowed with a plurality of favorable qualities and exposures which other patients do not happen to have in the same degree. The question is: Does randomization control for all these other shifting influences? In other words, have all sources of variance been exhausted to such a degree that only the treatment itself is responsible for differentiating responders from nonresponders? A pretrial evaluation of the patient by the physician on a basis of subjective assessment may prove useful in resolving this, and the question becomes: Does the physician's intuition, which I claim may be a valid procedural resource, lend itself to partitioning in such a way that his experience and understanding can be shared?

Collaborative Trials

Reasons for cooperation in trials by several institutions are twofold:

1. To provide a large enough combined sample to reveal true differences in response to one treatment and another, and
2. To involve all these institutions in a common educational experience.

In planning a cooperative trial, a leadership group with representatives from all involved institutions devises a common protocol, or flow plan. Every institution is supposed to follow this set of instructions point by point, in sequence, and without departures. A master randomization plan is used for casefinding and for the assignment of patients to experimental groups. Endpoints are commonly decided, statistical procedures are predicted and the least number of patients is specified for the entire trial, and for each institution. Details of time-dose radiotherapeutic relationships, surgery, and adjuvant therapies are determined. Normally, a central statistical facility is established where all data are funnelled.

A recent example of standard clinical trials by randomization, testing two treatment courses by protocol, is the preliminary report by the Committee for Radiation Studies, National Cancer Institute, in the February 1969 issue of CANCER [2], on preoperative irradiation for cancer of the lung. Seventeen medical centers cooperated in two separate trials of primary pulmonary carcinoma over a period of three years. A committee was established at each institution, consisting of surgeon, radiologist, and pathologist, and all data were sent to a statistical center for processing and analysis. Histological material was sent to a pathology center. Each patient was registered with the statistical center, evaluated clinically, and classified into one of three groups: Initially operable, potentially operable but with regional tissue invasion, and not suitable for resection (excluded).

The initially operable patients were randomly assigned to receive immediate surgery or preop radiotherapy and surgery, both groups in equal numbers. The surgical procedure was determined by the location of tumor, so we know that not all tumors were situated similarly. The potentially operable patients were also randomly assigned to receive surgery without additional therapy (except in the case of recurrence), or radiotherapy only. All patients were recalled every three months for an examination during the first year, and every six months thereafter.

An involved procedure was maintained to insure randomness, with lists maintained at each statistical center. Every new patient was reported to the statistical center by telephone for assignment. Of more than 3600 patients with primary cancer of the lung registered at the statistical center, only 16% met the criteria for the initially operable group and 12% were potentially operable, so it took a great many patients to achieve some kind of satisfactory sampling. In this way four randomized groups were obtained, with randomization effective for age, sex, color, degrees of disability, coincidental diseases, histologic type, and anatomic site of tumor, vital capacity and expiratory volume, nine variables. The authors of this first report make tabular comparisons to show that the samples were alike for all these variables, but there are percentage differences which could alter results. The results are not important, and I might add, nonsignificant. Survival was the endpoint, and differences for all groups were negligible. This is an ongoing project and the full work has yet to be reported, but it is a good example of how institutions can work together.

Roles of Participants

Neither the statistician nor the biometrician is necessarily a designer of trials. Designing an experimental plan is a philosophical exercise in logic and reason, a combination of art and science. The physician who requires insight into the effect of a treatment necessarily must be the artist who designs the procedure, and I would suggest that he use the statistician as he would a lawyer, to consult.

The statistician is indispensable in helping you to answer questions like: How big a caseload do I need to detect differences upon a level of significance providing faith in what I have found? How can I set up my data for best possible treatment? Given a maximum of competing patients, how can I best randomize them into two treatment groups and assess differences which may be meaningful? And, of course, he will do the calculations.

The biometrician sometimes can provide a mathematical basis for insights into data. Usually this has little application to clinical trials unless new designs are posed.

Statistical Treatments

Your choice of statistical comparisons will depend upon your original design. There is no point in discussing these things here because these are technicalities your statistician will be able to handle. For conventional designs you have a choice of retrospection, simple randomization, or stratified randomized designs, all with the usual tests for significance of differences upon some acceptable level. If you venture into some of the other designs that are being tried today, such as sequential analysis, matched-pair studies, or multivariate programs, you will need other statistical treatments.

Comparative Animal Studies

The relevance of trials with animals is related to the distance the experimental species is removed from humans. In general, results from animal trials are not easily extrapolable to humans because the distribution of specific tumors differs for every species, and also because humans are subject to variables which do not necessarily characterize captive animals. I have prepared Table I to show you some of the differences between animals and humans with regard to experimental programs. Aside from the fact that laboratory conditions are fixed, variables are known and controlled, and confidence in results can be maximally secure with a minimum of complications. The primary purpose of setting up animal experiments is to establish hypotheses which lend themselves to human explorations. This applies mostly to trials in the evaluation of two competitive treatments, not to experiments involving the induction of tumors. Also, ethical limitations upon human work are not present with animals. Animal designs are simpler than human because there is opportunity to work with genetically homozygous strains, as compared to panmixed humans, but this also can be a disadvantage because results are even more removed from human comparison. Since animal trials have been pursued for a long time, the literature is extensive, especially with regard to irradiation alone and in combination with surgery and chemotherapy. One other advantage in working with animals is that time is collapsed for all events, including the time from application of therapy to the endpoint. But results still are not easily extrapolated to humans, and in any event, endpoints such as the return of the individual to his life style cannot be considered.

The Partitioning of Intuition :
Pluralities of Variables Possibly Influencing End Results

SCHNEIDERMAN describes the power of 'subjective' judgment by the physician in predicting response in the cancer patient. While admitting the advantages of objective measures such as survival, he argues that objectivity leads to the selection of arbitrary endpoints which really are not the most suitable in terms of meaning-

Table I. Comparison of animal with human experimental designs

Trials	Animal	Human
Conditions	Relatively fixed	Fluid
Variables	Few, known, controlled	Many, some unknown, relatively uncontrolled
Experimental designs	Simple, especially with homozygous strains	Complex, to reduce bias and error
Statistical treatments	Usually simple, few, anticipated by design	Complex, many alternatives, subject to inference and interpretation
Usefulness of cooperative instrument (protocol)	None. Large populations available. Objectives are different.	Indispensable for cooperative projects, provides basis for reproducibility, assures adequate samples, uniformity and credibility.
Confidence in results	Secure, small differences detectable	Insecure even with large samples and extreme levels of significance. Small differences elusive.
Complicating factors	Survival of animals; questionable extrapolation of results to humans	Elimination of contributing bias; interactions and residual influence of known and unknown inborn and external variables; establishment of endpoints; sufficiently large samples; adequate trial designs; ethical considerations; followup and reproducibility of results; control of all participants and steps of trials, many others.
Objectives	Set up hypotheses which may be acceptable for human trials; search for hazards and side effects; preliminary studies of competing treatments.	Investigate alternative treatments for improved effect on disease; establish reasonable endpoints and measures for estimates of improvement; endow trials with highest possible degree of credibility and reproducibility.
Negative aspects; questions	Usefulness of results for human applications. Are species most used too far removed from humans? Are lab species subject to all the internal and external forces as are humans? Has the literature developed enough useful material to warrant large efforts in this direction?	Ethical limitations; time limitations; loss of patients from experiment; departures from designs and protocols; discontinuation by institutions; first and second type 'errors'; failure to explore influence of all possible variables upon endpoints. What is a reasonably human-oriented endpoint? Usefulness of medical intuition in predicting response or nonresponse. Many others.

ful evaluation. He further shows that the regression of a tumor is not necessarily correlated with survival rates, and his conclusion is that perhaps *total* patient response (increased wellbeing) without reference to length of survival or tumor shrinkage, is an improved and advanced basis for measurement.

I would like to substitute the word 'intuitive' for 'subjective', and to suggest that the intuition of the physician, while subjective and obscure, can be taken apart in such a way that some of the cues he senses in assessing the probability and degree of response on the part of his patient can be uncovered. In doing this, what we may be attempting is to discover those variables and interactions which can interfere with randomization, alone or in linked groups, and which can disturb variance to a sufficient extent that differences between two groups of treated cancer patients are either lost or falsely found. The methodology that exists for doing this is called *multivariate analysis*.

It never is easy to explain the rationale of multivariation. Picture all possible events in a clinical trial as analogous to a soup of different inorganic elements. It would be simple by assay to identify each element and its concentration. First you would decide what you want to find, and then you would decide how to find it, but you would guard against interference with your plan by combinations which might obscure results. How you would perform your assay is important. You could use wet methods with reagents. This tedious procedure would tell you that one ion at a time is present. You might want to use X-ray fluorescence to get about half a dozen elements at a time, but they would have to be reasonably heavy. Or, you could resort to spectroscopy and find all contained elements at the same time, and in relative concentrations. Now, if you made a matrix, like a map of road distances, lining up all elements across the top of a table, and also along the sides, you might be able to work out all possible interactions between all elements, and you might understand your soup. A computer could do all this for you, and even group ions that interact together, if properly programmed.

With clinical trials you have at least two groups of patients, and each is a competing soup. You have two treatments, and you measure their effectiveness by some kind of a predictable end result. You hope randomization obediently distributes all variables in your soups, so both are equivalent for every ingredient, but you quake in terror lest this doesn't work out. You have no way to assay for the presence of all components, and there are many such – molecular, cellular, hormonal, immunologic, genetic, and other inborn variables; plus external adaptations, exposures, influences, and fortuitous events during the patient's whole lifetime, during the treatment itself, and after the treatment in the interval reaching to the endpoint. All are interacting.

So you say, even if I find a fair percentage difference between two treatments, I can't believe what I find; or if I don't find such a reliable difference, maybe it was covered by some of these other influences. In Table II I have listed just 40 of all influences which could possibly have a bearing on your result. Some of these may be what physicians intuitively employ when they appraise a patient with respect to his degree of response to a given treatment.

You could at least list all possible variables in this universe and make a matrix. This is your assay. Most multivariate analyses are based on such a matrix where every variable is compared against each of the other variables. Often correlation coefficients are calculated. Then they can be coherently grouped. If all parameters could be controlled, if you could control the genetic bias, all host biases, all environmental influences, everything, then you wouldn't need protocols or flow sheets. You simply would randomize, stratifying only by those variables you can't control – age, race, sex, and pathologic comparability. Then you would administer radiotherapy by different time-dosage, or alternate surgical intervention and competing ionizing radiation, and that would do it. Clear results, more patients return to a useful life quickly, more survive longer thereafter, the tumor shrinks if it is solid; or else you find no differences and you make a decision. You can believe what you have found. But nothing works out this way. Even with other medical problems it never is easy. Some people seem to pick up viruses, others are resistant. Some people smoke for 70 years and nothing happens, others get one cancer or another, or a heart attack too early in life, or emphysema. And with treatments some are responders and others are nonresponders, some modalities work, others do not.

There are several alternative multivariate designs, and I will simply mention a few. Little clinical trial work has been done with

Table II. Some factors possibly contributing to variance in cancer clinical trials

Host Response (Responder–nonresponder)

Age
Race
Anatomic site of tumor
Histopathology: size, tissue type, stage of tumor
Immune response
Genetic factors
Concurrent pathology (esp. pathogenicity)
Preceding pathologic events
Personality factors
Hormonal levels
Environmental exposures and modifiers
Pre- and post-trial stresses

Treatment procedure

Dosage size and pattern
Time, duration and interval of doses
Single or combined modalities: Radiotherapy, surgery, chemotherapy
Adjuvant and palliative medication

External influences

Controlled sampling (randomization)
Design of trial (adequacy)
Rigor of protocol adherance: Departures, changes
Attitude of physician toward patients, personnel
Skill of medical operator: Surgery, radiology
Attitudes of nurses and other personnel toward patients
Team cooperation (medical interattitudinal variation)
Adequacy of record systems
Accuracy and integrity in following design
Time of day, month, year
Weather (temperature, humidity)
Place of trials
Replacement of personnel
Post-trial rehabilitation
Outlook for meaningful existence after trials ('Will to survive')
Sociocultural derivation

Analytic, procedural

Data keeping (uniform, adequate)
Sample size (adequacy)
Validation of patients as subjects
Randomization
Analysis of data

Other

Interactions of each of these variables with all others.
Interaction of groups of these variables with endpoints, as survival.
Competition or collaboration of groups of variables for residual variance.

any of these, and as far as I know factoring and clustering have never been tried. BULBROOK [1] has done some work with *discriminant functions,* working with breast cancers, and their response to adrenalectomy or hypophysectomy. A discriminant function is a classification measure. It fits a patient to a class of responders or nonresponders by a comparison, in this case relative excretion of two steroids. MACMAHAN [8] followed with a model for the use of multiple discriminant functions, and procedures for the identification of discriminants, and their usefulness. This kind of analysis is very complicated and you would require an expert to work with you.

To return to methods of clustering and factoring, this is the soup, or matrix, where you have listed all possible variables which could have an effect upon your endpoint. Any of these can contribute effectively to total variance, alone or with some of the others. If you knew all possible variables, and you could partition variance so well that you knew how effective each one was, you could at least reconsider your results, or accept them in good faith. Before you make your matrix you can take each variable and make a simple univariate comparison between both groups to see if they really are equivalent.

Now you have a matrix, all variables are compared, and there are systems that put these together in content-coherent groups. It is now possible to estimate how much each group contributes to total variance of the end result. If none produces much, your result becomes ascribable to your choice of treatment, and you can believe what you have found. If some of these variables seem to influence your result at least you can control for these in followup studies, or you can adjust for this additional variance and still find positive credibility.

In planning such a procedure you will need:

1. A list of all possible factors or variables, such as I have shown you.
2. A uniform trial design to which there is rigorous adherence by all.
3. Careful data designed into your procedure:
   a. Uniform laboratory procedures and report forms.
   b. A full questionnaire to be administered before, during, and after treatment. I learned recently that the Zellerbach-Saroni

Institute proposed RMP coding system has already taken steps in this direction, working from the Cantril model.
4. A method of treating the data.
5. A multivariationist who has worked in the philosophy and the implementation of multiple relationships in research. There really is no point in taking detailed data on many variables, and then drowning in your soup.

Now, if you cluster your universe of factors into primary variables upon each of which secondary (moderating) variables can operate, and you relate these groups to your criterion variable (the endpoint), you can see that there are all kinds of opportunity for interaction. If one primary variable is *radiation dose,* secondary moderating variables might be the sex of the patient, hormonal levels, immunologic response, genetic modifiers, age, physical condition, psychological assessment, and many others. Some of these would also operate upon other primary variables, say radiation time and interval. You might set up a cluster with preoperative surgery as the primary variable, and perhaps another with chemotherapy as adjuvant. You could have any number of these clusters of factors, and you could also have individual variables out by themselves because they do not modify any of these primary variables strongly enough to be included in clusters, yet they bear relationship to several, perhaps all. It can become quite complicated.

However, if you could determine the correlation of each cluster with the endpoint, you might be able to estimate how much each group of variables influences that endpoint, and what role each defining variable plays within each cluster. There are techniques for doing this with partial correlations, and also for determining how much each of these clusters contributes to total variance. When it is all over, you may find that most of your clusters disappear, leaving one treatment alone, or several in combination, as the truly meaningful influences upon the endpoint. In short, you might find that one or two definers (factors) in a cluster are pivotal, and that this cluster exerts most of the influence upon the endpoint. Then you can confidently feel you have preserved the full effect of randomization. Or else, you might find that some unsuspected factors, perhaps psychological status or immune response or differential hormonal levels, contribute more to the effect than you could anticipate if you hadn't taken this data and analyzed it, and you might have to alter the treatment or run new trials.

Conclusion

The problem is simple. You have randomized a group of patients into two separate subgroups, each of which will receive a competing treatment, one of which is standard. Your statistician tells you how big a sample you must have to be reasonably secure upon apreselected level of statistical confidence, how much improvement is convincing, or what percentage of cases should show as a difference between both groups. It is assumed you have chosen an endpoint, or several, the obvious ones of which are survival rates, tumor shrinkage, and recurrence. Another endpoint might be the return of the patient to a useful life.

The statistician is correct in his rationale, but there are some simple additional statements you can make: (1) If you controlled for obvious influences, and if you eliminated all other variables, then *any* excess of improvement in the experimental group is worth pursuing. (2) It is by no means secure that randomization will distribute all variables uniformly in two competing populations. The nature of variability is such that if you have enough variables, these can accumulate unevenly in any population that isn't extremely large. Also, there is the role of the clinician as a 'guesser' who evaluates each patient as a prospective responder, and there are interactions of the total environment following treatment before the endpoint can occur.

Some of the unknown variance which may condition results is 'felt' intuitively by the physician who subjectively assesses his patients from long experience. Multivariate treatments attempt to look into this residual variance, and into intuition, by defining all possible sources of error or bias, naming them, exploring them, and finding out how much they contribute to the endpoint.

Nothing in life is univariate, no variable is an island unto itself, and randomization controls only insofar as you can be sure other influences have not interfered with an accurate appraisal of results. If small differences between two groups of treated patients are at stake, it is especially important to drop out all possible sources of influence other than the treatments themselves.

Multiple variables can be programmed at the beginning of clinical trials, and especially in cooperative trials, in order to increase our confidence. In doing this, laboratory procedures and questionnaires should be carefully designed and followed. All possible physiologic discriminating events which could influence response should be established. Additionally, all possible external influences which could affect the success or failure of a trial should be probed with a structured questionnaire. Resulting data should be analysed to determine contributions of each set of variables to the endpoint. In this way we will not only partition the physician's 'non-objective' appraisal, but we will be providing a system that can be used for replication.

References

1. BULBROOK, R. D. and HAYWOOD, J. L.: Endocrine studies in patients with early breast cancer; in Current concepts in breast cancer, pp. 115–131 (Williams & Wilkins, Baltimore 1967).
2. Committee for Radiation Studies, National Cancer Institute, NIH, PHS: Preoperative irradiation of cancer of the lung. Cancer, 23 : 419–429 (1969).
3. CORNFIELD, J.: Tentative design of a cooperative experiment; in KAPLAN Research in radiology (National Academy of Sciences, National Research Council, Washington 1958).
4. DEELEY, T. J.: Controlled clinical trials in radiotherapy; in VAETH Frontiers in radiation therapy and oncology, vol. 2 (Karger, Basel/München/New York 1968).
5. FISHER, R. A.: Statistical methods for research workers. FAE Crew (Oliver & Boyd, Edinburgh 1948).
6. KELLER, A. R.; KAPLAN, H. S.; LUKES, R. J., and RAPPAPORT, H.: Correlation of histopathology with other prognostic indicators in Hodgkin's disease. Cancer 22 : 487–499 (1968).
7. LARIONOV, L. F.: Cancer chemotherapy (Pergamon Press, Oxford 1965).
8. McMAHAN, C. A.: Empirical effects of measurement error on a two-variable discriminant function based on urinary steroids; in Current concepts in breast cancer, pp. 151–186 (Williams & Wilkins, Baltimore 1967).
9. SCHNEIDERMAN, M. A.: Non-objective art and objective evaluation in cancer chemotherapy; in BRODSKY and KAHN Cancer chemotherapy. The 15th Hahnemann Symposium (Grune & Stratton, New York 1967).
10. WATSON, I. A.: Clinical trials in a radiotherapy center. Cancer 22 : 711–715 (1968).

Author's address: Dr. I. D. ROTKIN, Department of Preventive Medicine and Community Health, The University of Illinois, Medical Center, Chicago, IL 60680 (USA).

Discussion

Moderator:

DONALD G. BAKER, Ph. D., Head, Division of Oncologic and Radiobiologic Research, Claire Zellerbach Saroni Tumor Institute, *San Francisco, Calif.*

Discussant:

ROBERT F. KALLMAN, Ph. D., Chief, Radiology Research; Associate Professor of Radiology, Stanford University School of Medicine, *Palo Alto, Calif.*

KALLMAN: Having listened to the five papers presented this morning and having already read the complete manuscripts of these papers, I am supposed to discuss them by coordinating what the various speakers have said, bringing out points of controversy, or perhaps by presenting additional material which might either confirm or contradict evidence that you have heard. I hope this won't disappoint anyone, but I am afraid that I find it impossible to do most of these things. The papers we have heard cover an extremely wide range of questions – from fundamental cellular radiobiology in the laboratory to clinical trials with patients, and it seems to me that all of the speakers have made their points effectively and concisely. Also, as I myself have not been concerned, experimentally, with the immediate subject of preoperative radiotherapy, I cannot introduce additional data into the discussion.

However, it seems to me that one thing comes through rather strongly. Of course I may be prejudiced in bringing this out and I may be deluded by my own position or interests, but I believe that it is true that much of the impetus for undertaking preoperative radiotherapy as a treatment modality stems from the advances that have been made in the laboratory in cellular radiobiology. In fact, it might even be correct to claim that the entire effort came about as the direct result of concepts that have emerged from laboratory studies using material ranging from bacterial cells to mouse tumor cells. I think it is important to bring this out, in view of the fact that we radiobiologists frequently hear the radiotherapist say, 'these radiobiology experiments in the laboratory are very interesting, but what have they told us that will help solve the pressing clinical problems that we have to confront constantly?'

As Dr. PEREZ pointed out at the beginning of this morning's session, the central reason for using preoperative radiotherapy is to kill as many cancer cells as possible prior to surgery, thereby reducing the risk of dissemination that might otherwise have a high probability with a large tumor mass. Survival curves that have been produced with a variety of cells in the laboratory have convinced many people that fairly modest doses which might be inadequate to cure the tumor, do have the effect of substantially reducing the cell population – up to several orders of magnitude. That this kind of theoretical reasoning is sound is borne out by trials, both in the laboratory and clinic, as we shall hear further in the papers to be presented after this morning.

Dr. BELLI has summarized for us some of the basic radiobiological factors that must be taken into account in the optimization of preoperative radiotherapy. As he has pointed out, it is essential that one be aware of the kinetics of the repair of radiation damage in order that, for example, one might be able intelligently to choose the best timing of irradiation and surgery. Dr. BELLI's remarks were addressed primarily to how this choice should be made with respect to the cells of the tumor which is to be removed surgically. I should simply like to add that the kinetics of injury repair are of at least equal importance for the normal tissues that are inevitably included in the radiation field and that are of paramount importance in the healing of the surgical field. Therefore, I think we should all be aware of the fact that the repair of sub-lethal or potentially lethal injury in *normal* cells must be taken into account in deriving a better understanding of this whole subject. I think it is correct to say that the repair kinetics of both kinds of cells, normal and malignant, do not differ qualitatively, so that what Dr. BELLI has told us and emphasized as important for the tumor is just as valid for the normal cells. If we have time, I think it would be useful if Dr. BELLI would comment on this.

Dr. PEREZ has provided us with a most thorough discussion of the theoretical basis of preoperative radiotherapy, the experimental evidence which should be brought to bear in utilizing this modality in the clinic, and some important questions that remain to be answered. Although he was unable to present his complete manuscript in the session this morning, I can assure you that his paper, which will appear in the published proceedings of this meeting, is quite comprehensive. For reasons that I think Dr. PEREZ has made amply clear, his extensive laboratory work and that of his collaborators has been done with an experimental tumor system which, while it lends itself extremely well to this kind of investigation, has certain shortcomings in its applicability to many of the situations that have to be dealt with clinically. The 6C3HED lymphosarcoma is indeed a convenient tumor to work with experimentally and, historically, it has provided us, in the hands of POWERS and TOLMACH, with some of the most basic information we have about *in vivo* tumor radiobiology. Nonetheless, one must keep in mind the fact that this tumor is a lymphosarcoma, it is distinctly antigenic, and its cells are killed by radiation by a mechanism which may not be typical of that experienced by the cells of many other tumors, for example, carcinomas and other kinds of sarcomas. Therefore, I believe we have to join with Dr. PEREZ in hoping that others will undertake parallel studies in, hopefully, a variety of other tumor systems. Most of us who work in the laboratory tend to focus our attention upon a single experimental system, simply because there is not sufficient time to survey other systems. We are aware of the limitations about what we may be fortunate enough to discover, and we all hope that we personally will find time to extend our work to other kinds of tumors or systems – a hope that is all too often unrealized – or that other interested colleagues might be encouraged to do this. We have seen, in Dr. INCH's paper, an example of the importance of tumor growth rate on the effectiveness of preoperative radio-therapy. Even with a population of tumors all of the same type and all derived from the same donor tissue, one may see a clear example of heterogeneity of treatment response: slower growing tumors are more effectively treated than fast growing tumors. In this case, we are fortunate that it is possible to correlate local recurrence rate with tumor growth rate.

Dr. PEREZ has enumerated for us several parameters of preoperative irradiation and has discussed them in detail – the optimal dose of radiation, the optimal time between irradiation and surgery, the effects of radiation dose fractionation, the value of adjuvant chemotherapy and immunotherapy, and the effects of preoperative irradiation on wound healing. In his manuscript, he introduced one thought that I found intriguing: the advantage – theoretically at least – of a preoperative radiation course given as two fractions. The first fraction would serve primarily to bring about shrinkage of the tumor and the second fraction would be given largely to maximize tumor cell killing. Shrinkage is important not only to facilitate surgical excision of a more manageable tumor mass, but in order to bring about improved tumor oxygenation so that further irradiation will in fact kill more cells. Of course, this raises the whole question of optimization of the strategy of fractionation, and this has been the subject of an earlier San Francisco Cancer Symposium [1967], as well as other symposia, notably the one that was held just last month in Carmel. I don't propose to deal with this at length, except to say that perhaps the problems to be met in preoperative radiotherapy may be, in this respect, less complex than those confronting the radiotherapist who is attempting to get tumor control or cure by radiation alone. Perhaps, in preoperative radiotherapy, the therapist can afford to follow the volume of the lesion more closely after, say, an initial large dose, and could thereby choose the best time for the second of two doses that might constitute the entire preoperative course. Tumors behave differently after an initial radiation dose, some continue to grow and some shrink promptly, so the optimal timing of two doses may well be variable from tumor to tumor; it could range from around a day to perhaps a week or two between doses. Possibly, this line of reasoning betrays my naïveté, for I speak as a radiobiologist. But perhaps it is not so naïve and it might bear serious consideration for its practical applicability.

I was interested in Dr. INCH's findings that preoperative radiotherapy was more effective if the dose was delivered 6 days as compared to 1 or 12 days prior to surgery. To me, this is consistent with the reasoning that I just voiced. Dr. INCH was concerned with the state of the tumor at the time of surgery; that is, the experiments were not designed to study the relative effectiveness of fractionated irradiation. But the same considerations would hold: the tumor should be more responsive to a second dose of radiation at 6 days, so for this tumor the optimum fractionation interval might be relatively long. In the case of Dr. PEREZ' tumor, surgery was more effective when performed 1 or 3 days after irradiation, as contrasted with a 7 day interval. Unfortunately, Dr. PEREZ does not have experimental data to bear on the two-fraction radiation idea, and his multiple fraction data are not sufficient to answer this question.

Dr. GOLDMAN has presented some interesting evidence and I think that some of this evidence bears further investigation or perhaps reinvestigation. I refer to the work he reported with tritiated thymidine. This certainly represents a valiant attempt at disclosing viable remaining tumor cells. It is relevant to inquire, however, whether the technique used to introduce the thymidine into the cells was adequate. STEEL and his collaborators in England have developed a technique designed to overcome the incomplete perfusion of a biopsy specimen by tritiated thymidine when the specimen is simply placed in a medium containing the labeled compound. The technique involves the generation of many atmospheres of pressure within a small pressure bomb. Even under these conditions, labeling patterns obtained *in vitro* have been found by Steel and many others not to resemble the patterns obtained in the same animal tumors *in vivo*. Primarily for this reason, the labeling described by Dr. GOLDMAN may have little quantitative validity although it certainly remains a valuable qualitative demonstration of the fact that DNA synthesis is going on in these irradiated cells. But here we must keep in mind still one further reservation. It has been shown repeatedly in controlled laboratory experiments that cells which have been killed may, in fact, not die for considerable periods of time. Furthermore, such reproductively-killed cells would be expected to be entirely capable of synthesizing DNA, and therefore of incorporating tritiated thymidine, before they reach the critical mitotic division when they are likely to die. For this reason, one might question the validity of labeling indices obtained especially during the course of radiotherapy or even shortly after it has been completed.

I have really no constructive comment to make about Dr. ROTKIN's paper except to say that I consider it a most interesting and remarkably concise presentation of an enormously important subject. Clinical trials are the *sine qua non* of radiobiology and the clinician, in particular, should be aware of new advances and principles in their proper implementation. Indeed, we will hear about several clinical trials throughout the remainder of this symposium. But I was particularly taken with Dr. ROTKIN's advice about cooperative trials. Because I had chatted briefly with him some time ago and I had an idea of what he was going to say, I was especially interested to learn, at the Carmel meeting on dose fractionation, about the progress of the ongoing British Institute of Radiology fractionation study reported by Dr. F. ELLIS. At least to me, this study constitutes a prime example of how a well-designed cooperative trial can be carried out. I don't propose to deliver Dr. ELLIS' paper for him, and therefore I will make no attempt to cover all of the very important aspects of the BIR study. The study was designed to evaluate the effectiveness of radiotherapy delivered in 3 fractions per week *vs.* 5 fractions per week. Since the start of this study in 1966, 15 cooperating centers have contributed a total of 228 patients for treatment of cancers of the larynx and pharynx. The interim progress report just given us by Dr. ELLIS covers three and one-half years. At this stage of the program, there seems to be no significant difference between the effects of 3 fractions per week and 5 fractions per week on normal tissues or on tumors. I am not introducing this in the discussion because of the radiotherapeutic importance of the study. The conclusion about the absence of a difference is provisional. And, moreover, the subject is not really the overriding consideration of this symposium. I mention it primarily to illustrate that it is indeed possible to enlist the cooperation of a large number of otherwise independent clinicians in the investigation of a subject of great importance. Needless to say, I regard the design of the BIR study as superior, in that they apparently have taken into account all of the factors enumerated by Dr. ROTKIN.

Front. Radiation Ther. Onc., vol. 5, pp. 93–99
(Karger, Basel/München/Paris/New York 1970)

Radical Preoperative Radiation Therapy in Primarily Inoperable Advanced Cancers of the Oral Cavity[1]

M. GALANTE, S. BENAK, Jr., and F. BUSCHKE

University of California, San Francisco Medical Center; Department of Surgery and Cancer Research Institute, and Section of Therapeutic Radiology, Department of Radiology, University of California School of Medicine; San Francisco, Calif.

Considerable clinical work has been done during the past 15 years demonstrating unequivocally that extensive surgical procedures can be carried out in practically any organ system without increased morbidity or mortality following preoperative administration of X-ray therapy in significant doses [1, 2, 3, 4, 5]. Still, the misconception that the risk of operating in irradiated tissues is increased or prohibitive cannot be completely eradicated from the minds of many surgeons as well as radiation therapists. The persistence of this prejudice justifies the presentation of one phase of our experience with the use of preoperative radiation therapy and radical surgery for a number of lesions of the oral cavity.

The selection of a patient for this method of treatment cannot be scientifically infallible; it is a subjective process that depends almost entirely on the clinical judgment and experience of the clinicians involved in this decision. Host resistance, the biology and radiosensitivity of a particular tumor, the geographical limits of microscopic extent of tumor cells into surrounding tissues are but a few of many essential factors which we cannot properly assess and utilize at the present time for a more objective selection of these patients. This selection is determined entirely by previous clinical observation; patients who are thought to be highly curable by surgery alone or by radiation therapy alone are excluded from this plan.

[1] This investigation was supported in part by NIH Grant CA 5177, National Cancer Institute, National Institutes of Health.

Patients selected for integrated treatment fall essentially into two groups: (a) Patients with primary lesions usually treated surgically but of such size as to make it impossible to resect them with adequate tumor-free margins. This group constitutes the majority of patients. (b) Patients with lesions that are too differentiated or too invasive into bone, muscle or lymph nodes for control by radiation therapy alone.

Three factors must be considered in the administration of radiation therapy to patients considered for the combined treatment: (a) the total dose; (b) the total time and fractionation; (c) the optimal interval between irradiation and surgery.

Total Dose

It is assumed that it is impossible to assess clinically in patients the biological effect of radiation therapy on individual cancer cells and their ability to implant and grow as distant metastases when and if such cells are freed into the circulation during surgical manipulations of a tumor. It is also assumed that there is no way to measure in patients any deleterious or beneficial systemic effects of radiations on host resistance. Therefore, for practical purposes, the effect of radiations on the gross tumor itself is the only change that can be clinically evaluated. Thus, a total dose ordinarily considered to be sufficient for maximal reduction of the size of the lesion with the least damage to the surrounding tissues is utilized, i.e., 5,000 to 6,500 rads/tumor dose delivered in 6 to 7 weeks (NSD = 1,400 to 1,600 rets) (table I). Although it is fully realized that this may constitute an oversimplification of the problem, the aim of this plan has been *to convert an inoperable into an operable lesion by sheer diminution of the bulk of the primary tumor,* thus increasing the surgical margins of uninvolved tissue without necessarily sterilizing the most resistant central region of the tumor.

Total Time and Fractionation

The experience reported by BACLESSE [1] showed clearly the advantage of protracting therapy for several weeks, increasing the differential between the vulnerability of neoplastic and normal tissues sufficiently to cure advanced carcinomas even with medium-volt therapy. By utilizing this technique in conjunction with high-energy radiation such as ^{60}Co radiation, the damage to the vasculo-connective tissue, so essential in reparative and healing processes, is minimized. Our experience indicates that the protraction of therapy over 6 to 7 weeks, with the administration of 900 rads tumor dose per week, produces minimal reaction of the soft tissues with satisfactory reduction of the size of the tumor (table I).

Since the primary aim of radiation therapy is to sterilize the peripheral portion of the disease, the fields utilized must be large enough to include the primary tumor with adequate surrounding margins of grossly normal tissue, as well as the immediately adjacent lymph nodes, particularly if the latter are suspected to be clinically involved. Ordinarily for lesions of the oral cavity no attempt is made to treat the entire neck area.

Table I. Method of preoperative irradiation

A)	Equipment	1.	1 MeV G.E. Maxitron, HVL 3.2 mm lead
		2.	Theratron F Cobalt-60, HVL 11 mm lead
B)	Dose	5,000–6,500 rads/tumor dose	
C)	Time	6–7 weeks (900 rads/tumor dose per week)	
		(NSD = 1,400–1,600 rets)	
D)	Volume	Primary region with adequate margin and adjacent palpable nodes	

Interval between Radiation and Surgery

The selection of the 'optimal' time for surgery is greatly influenced by the fact that the authors do not consider cancer, especially epitheliomas of the oral cavity, a surgical emergency, particularly after the lesions have been treated with a significant dose of radiation.

The selection of time for operation depends on the observed response of the tumor during and following therapy, as well as the condition of the irradiated tissues.

Experience has shown that the best criterion for determining the optimal time for surgery is observation of the patient at weekly intervals until maximum shrinkage of the tumor is accompanied by maximum regression of tissue reaction (mucositis, edema, erythema); surgery however should not be delayed to the point where the reparative processes may have produced a significant degree of fibrosis. Experience has also shown that one is more likely to err by operating prematurely rather than by delaying the operation too long. For example, the degree of fibrosis encountered in one patient operated five and one-half months following completion of X-ray therapy was not sufficient to create significant technical difficulties during operation nor to impair the healing of mucosa, soft tissues and skin in any way. With a few individual variations, most patients appear to be ready for operation sometime between the sixth and the twelfth week after the completion of therapy, when the reaction of irradiated tissues is at a minimum and systemic recovery of the patient at a maximum.

The operative procedure employed is always a combined resection of the primary lesion en bloc with the regional cervical lymph nodes so as to obtain a continuous specimen which includes tongue, tonsillar pillars, floor of the mouth, hemimandible, as required by the location of the primary lesion, with the contents of a standard homolateral radical neck dissection. No 'modification' of the combined resection is employed; *radiation therapy is administered to increase the margins of normal tissue resected, not to decrease the extent and scope of the operation.*

Unless a tumor proves to be unexpectedly radiosensitive and regresses to suggest that complete control will be obtained by irradiation alone, surgery is performed. Post-radiation biopsies are not obtained regardless of the local findings because a biopsy specimen is not an infallible test for tumor cells or for their biological potential.

During the decade 1957–1966, 29 patients with lesions considered too large for primary surgery or not suitable for radiation therapy alone were treated by integrated radiation therapy and radical surgery (table II).

It is impossible to make any conclusions regarding survival with such a small group of patients beyond stating that the results appear to indicate that the 2- and 5-year tumor-free survival rates are significant in a group of patients with lesions ordinarily considered unfavorable and uncontrollable by radical surgery or radiotherapy alone (table III).

Examination of the specimens indicated that the surgical excision was always microscopically beyond the margins of the tumor and that in 4 cases there was no evidence of disease at the primary site or in the lymph nodes (table IV).

Table II

Site of lesion	Number of patients
Anterior pillar	11
Palate	1
Alveolar ridge	3
Buccal mucosa	1
Floor of mouth	7
Oral tongue	6
Total	29

Table III

Site of lesion	2-Year determinate survival	5-Year determinate survival
Anterior pillar	7/11 (63.6%)	5/7 (71.4%)
Palate	1/1 (100%)	—
Alveolar ridge	3/3 (100%)	—
Buccal mucosa	0/1	—
Floor of mouth	4/7 (57.1%)	2/3 (66.7%)
Oral tongue	1/6 (16.7%)	0/5

Table IV. Pathology of surgical specimens

Site of lesion	Primary site +	Primary site −	Nodes +	Nodes −
Anterior pillar	8	3	2	9
Palate	0	1	0	1
Alveolar ridge	3	0	1	2
Buccal mucosa	1	0	0	1
Floor of mouth	7	0	4	3
Oral tongue	6	0	5	1

Table V. Complications following combined treatment

Fibrosis	4
Suture sinus	1
Skin flap necrosis	1
Salivary fistula	4

The number and nature of complications occurring post-operatively in irradiated tissues were not serious and did not vary from those associated with similar surgical procedures performed in non-irradiated tissues (table V). Four minor salivary fistulae healed spontaneously without operative intervention. Grossly noticeable fibrosis was encountered in 4 patients without producing significant technical difficulties at the time of operation. One patient developed a 3×4 cm area of skin necrosis requiring a skin graft for complete healing of the wound. Removal of a deeply located nonabsorbable suture in another patient was followed by spontaneous healing of a chronically draining sinus.

The main purpose of this presentation is to emphasize that radical surgery is feasible in previously irradiated tissues with technical operative features, morbidity and complications comparable to those of similar operations performed in nonirradiated tissues.

As stated in a previous publication [5], '...surgery and radiation therapy are not competitive or mutually exclusive. The well-planned utilization of both disciplines can be of great help in the management of properly selected cases. But the most important single prerequisite for this kind of radical management is complete mutual understanding and close cooperation between surgeon and radiotherapist in planning prior to treatment and throughout its entire course, with repeated re-evaluation of the response of the disease and of the tolerance of normal tissues, and corresponding adjustment of the original plan during and following irradiation.'

References

1. BACLESSE, F.: Clinical experience with ultra-fractionated roentgen therapy; in BUSCHKE Progress in radiation therapy, vol. 1, chap. 6 (Grune and Stratton, New York 1958).

2. BRONSTEIN, E. L.; HUSTU, O.; CLIFFTON, E. E., and GOODNER, J. T.: Preoperative irradiation in the treatment of cancer of the esophagus. Reported at the meeting of the Radiological Society of North America, November, 1959.
3. BUSCHKE, F.: Common misconceptions in radiation therapy. Amer. J. Surg. *101*: 164–170 (1961).
4. BUSCHKE, F.; CANTRIL, S. T., and PARKER, H. M.: Supervoltage roentgentherapy (Thomas, Springfield 1950).
5. BUSCHKE, F. and GALANTE, M.: Radical preoperative roentgen therapy in primarily inoperable advanced cancers of the head and neck. Radiology *73*: 845–848 (1959).

Authors' addresses: Dr. MAURICE GALANTE, University of California, U-112, Radiology Department of Surgery and Cancer Research Institute, San Francisco Medical Center, *San Francisco, CA 94122* ; Dr. STEVE BENAK, Jr.; Dr. FRANZ BUSCHKE, Section of Therapeutic Radiology, Department of Radiology; University of California School of Medicine, *San Francisco, CA 94122* (USA).

Front. Radiation Ther. Onc., vol. 5, pp. 100–105
(Karger, Basel/München/Paris/New York 1970)

Planned Preoperative Irradiation for Laryngeal and Laryngopharyngeal Carcinoma

H. F. BILLER and J. H. OGURA

Department of Otolaryngology, Washington University School of Medicine, St. Louis, Mo.

Introduction

Clinical studies appear to indicate that planned preoperative irradiation increases survival for patients with large laryngeal and laryngopharyngeal cancers [2, 3, 4, 5]. These studies have examined small patient populations and the results, though appearing to confirm the efficacy of preoperative irradiation, are not statistically significant.

In a recent publication [1], the authors presented a retrospective study of 251 patients with laryngeal and laryngopharyngeal cancers treated with and without preoperative irradiation. This analysis indicated that preoperative irradiation increased the survival rate for patients with laryngopharyngeal cancers, but again the difference was not statistically significant. This paper includes an additional 41 patients, making a total of 292 cases for analysis. The variables investigated include 3-year survival, local recurrence, neck recurrence, and complications.

Preoperative Irradiation

The preoperative irradiation was administered, using ^{60}Co teletherapy units, 1,500 R to 3,000 R, over a two to three week period to the primary lesion and ipsilateral neck. Surgery was performed 3 to 4 weeks following the completion of radiation therapy. The surgical resection was determined by the extent of the lesion, prior to irradiation. An in-continuity neck dissection was performed, whether or not nodes were palpable.

Material and Methods

Five hundred and thirty-three cases of laryngeal and laryngopharyngeal cancers treated at McMillan Hospital, Washington University, from 1955 through August 1966 were reviewed. Two hundred and eight cases, representing glottic lesions treated by hemilaryngectomy or total laryngectomy, were excluded, due to the absence of a comparable group receiving preoperative irradiation. The remaining 325 cases were treated by partial or total laryngectomy with neck dissection. One hundred thirty-five of these cases received planned preoperative irradiation and 190 cases did not. Fifteen patients from the preoperative group and 18 patients from the non-preoperative group died of known intercurrent disease and are excluded from the study, resulting in 120 and 172 patients, respectively, for comparison.

The entire group of cases are considered homogenous and comparable, in that the cases were all examined, classified, and operated upon by one of us (JHO). Standard operating techniques were employed in both series.

The lesions were classified as supraglottic, transglottic, pyriform sinus, base of tongue and vallecula. The pathology records were used for this classification. Nodes were considered positive if there was histologic evidence of tumor.

Tumors which involved more than one area were classified with that tumor which has the greater incidence of metastatic disease. Therefore, laryngeal tumors which involve pharyngeal areas, are classified as pharyngeal lesions.

Results were compared for statistical significance by utilizing the Chi Square test in a 2×2 classification. A confidence level of 95% ($P = 0.05$) was considered statistically significant.

Results

Supraglottic Lesions – Table I

Supraglottic lesions involve the epiglottis and/or the false cords. A total of 87 cases are included; 35 received preoperative irradiation and 52 were treated without preoperative irradiation. The incidence of positive nodes is 15/35 (42%) and 17/52 (32%), respectively.

There is no significant difference between the two groups, for local recurrence, neck recurrence, or survival.

Transglottic Lesions – Table II

Transglottic lesions involve both true and false vocal cords. Seventy-three cases are included. Thirty received preoperative irradiation and 40 were treated without preoperative irradiation. The incidence of positive nodes is 12/30 (40%) and 17/43 (39%), respectively. There is no significant difference between the two groups, for survival, local recurrence, or neck recurrence.

Base of Tongue and Vallecular Lesions – Table III
These lesions involve the lingual surface of the epiglottis, vallecula and base of tongue posterior to the circumvallate papilla. Twenty-nine lesions are included. Fourteen received preoperative irradiation and 15 were treated without preoperative irradiation. The incidence of positive nodes is 10/14 (71%) and 8/15 (53%), respectively. There is no significant difference between the two groups for survival, local or neck recurrence.

Table I. Supraglottic lesions

	3-Year survival	Local recurrence	Neck recurrence	Distant metastases	Complications	Lost to follow-up
Preoperative irradiation	26/35 (74%)	1/35 (2.8%)	1/35 (2.8%)	6/35 (17%)	2/35 (5.7%)	1
No preoperative irradiation	45/52 (86%)	0/52 (0%)	2/52 (3.8%)	4/52 (7.6%)	2/52 (3.8%)	1

Table II. Transglottic lesions

	3-Year survival	Local recurrence	Neck recurrence	Distant metastases	Complications	Lost to follow-up
Preoperative irradiation	16/30 (53%)	3/30 (10%)	6/30 (20%)	2/30 (6.6%)	6/30 (20%)	3
No preoperative irradiation	30/43 (69%)	3/43 (6.9%)	4/43 (9%)	2/43 (4.6%)	6/43 (13%)	4

Table III. Base of tongue and vallecula lesions

	3-Year survival	Local recurrence	Neck recurrence	Distant metastases	Complications	Lost to follow-up
Preoperative irradiation	7/14 (50%)	0/14 (0%)	4/14 (28%)	2/14 (14%)	2/14 (14%)	1
No preoperative irradiation	6/15 (40%)	3/15 (20%)	5/15 (33%)	1/15 (6.6%)	1/15 (6.6%)	0

Pyriform Sinus Lesions – Table IV

A total of 103 cases are included. Forty-one received preoperative irradiation and 62 were treated without preoperative irradiation. The incidence of positive nodes is 29/41 (70%) and 48/63 (77%), respectively.

The results indicate a statistically significant ($X^2_c = 11.432$: $P = 0.0007$) increase in three-year survival rate for those patients treated with preoperative irradiation. There is no significant difference between the two groups for local or neck recurrence.

Laryngopharyngeal Lesions (Base of Tongue and Pyriform Sinus) – Table V

Combining the pharyngeal lesions (base of tongue and pyriform sinus), to obtain a larger population, results in a statistically significant decrease in local recurrence with preoperative irradiation ($X^2_c = 4.887$: $P = 0.027$).

Table IV. Pyriform sinus lesions

	3-Year survival	Local recurrence	Neck recurrence	Distant metastases	Complications	Lost to follow-up
Preoperative irradiation	25/41 (60%)	4/41 (9.7%)	7/41 (17%)	4/41 (9.7%)	3/41 (7.3%)	1
No preoperative irradiation	26/62 (41%)	15/62 (24%)	13/62 (20%)	1/62 (1.6%)	9/62 (14.5%)	7

$$(X^2_c = 11.432: P = 0.0007)$$

Table V. Base of tongue and pyriform sinus lesions

	3-Year survival	Local recurrence	Neck recurrence	Distant metastases	Complications	Lost to follow-up
Preoperative irradiation	32/55 (58%)	4/55 (7%)	11/55 (20%)	6/55 (10.9%)	5/55 (9%)	2
No preoperative irradiation	32/77 (41%)	18/77 (23%)	18/77 (23%)	2/77 (2.5%)	10/77 (13%)	7

$$(X^2_c = 4.887: P = 0.027)$$

Discussion

Preoperative irradiation as defined in this presentation does not affect all types of laryngeal lesions equally.

Preoperative irradiation had no influence on transglottic and supraglottic lesions in regard to survival, local recurrence or neck recurrence. If it is correct that preoperative irradiation destroys the well oxygenated peripheral cells, thereby leaving a small nucleus of viable central cells, it is not surprising that supraglottic and transglottic lesions are not influenced by preoperative irradiation. These cancers are usually adequately encompassed by the routine total laryngectomy for transglottic, and partial laryngectomy for transglottic, and partial laryngectomy for supraglottic lesions. The 0% local recurrence for supraglottic lesions and the 7% local recurrence for transglottic lesions, without preoperative irradiation, confirms the adequacy of the surgical procedure employed.

The adequacy of surgical margins is not as secure in pyriform sinus and base of tongue cancers. Tumor margins may be difficult to discern and submucosal involvement frequently occurs. If the theoretical rationale of preoperative irradiation is valid, a decrease in the incidence of local recurrence with pyriform sinus and base of tongue lesions should be expected and this should be reflected in an increased survival rate. This is suggested by the study. The number of base of tongue lesions in this series is too small to draw conclusions. Though the incidence of local recurrence of base of tongue cancers with preoperative irradiation was 0%, versus 20% without preoperative irradiation, the difference is not statistically significant ($X^2_{ch} = 1.339$: $P = 0.25$).

The pyriform sinus cancers indicate a trend toward decreased local recurrence with preoperative irradiation ($X^2_c = 2.527$: $P = 0.11$) and demonstrate a statistically significant increase in the three-year survival ($X^2_c = 11.432$: $P = 0.0007$).

Combining the two pharyngeal groups (base of tongue and pyriform sinus), in order to obtain a larger population, results in a statistically significant decrease in local recurrence with pre-operative irradiation ($X^2_c = 4.887$: $P = 0.027$). This is reflected in a trend toward increased survival ($X^2_c = 2.915$: $P = 0.08$).

Neck recurrence was not influenced by preoperative irradiation. This fact does not concur with the results reported by STRONG *et al.* [6] who indicate a decrease in neck recurrence with preoperative irradiation.

Strong's series consisted mainly of oropharyngeal lesions, rather than laryngeal, which may indicate that the response to irradiation of nodes of different primaries is not the same.

Complications evaluated in this series include fistula and skin slough requiring a graft. In no instance were complications increased by preoperative irradiation.

Summary

A retrospective study was performed in an attempt to evaluate the efficacy of low dose planned preoperative irradiation utilizing 1,500 R to 3,000 R, in the treatment of laryngeal and laryngopharyngeal cancer. It appears that low dose preoperative irradiation benefits only laryngopharyngeal cancers. Neck recurrence and complications were not influenced by preoperative irradiation.

References

1. BILLER, H. F.; OGURA, J. H.; DAVIS, W. H., and POWERS, W. E.: Planned preoperative irradiation for carcinoma of the larynx and laryngopharynx treated by total and partial laryngectomy. Laryngoscope (in press).
2. GOLDMAN, J. L.; SILVERSTONE, S. M.; ROSIN, H. D.; CHEREN, R. V., and ZAK, F. G.: Combined radiation and surgical therapy for cancer of the larynx and laryngopharynx. Laryngoscope *74:* 1,111–1,134 (1964).
3. HENDRICKSON, F. R. and LIEBNER, B.: Results of preoperative radiotherapy for supraglottic larynx cancer. Ann. Otol. Rhinol. Laryng., St. Louis *77:* 222–230 (1968).
4. SKOLNIK, E. M.; TENTA, L. T.; COMITO, J. M., and JEROME, D. L.: Preoperative radiation in head and neck cancer. Ann. Otol. Rhinol. Laryng., St. Louis *75:* 336–355 (1966).
5. SKOLNIK, E. M.; SOBOROFF, B. J.; TENTA, L. T.; SABERMAN, M. N., and Jones, H. C.: Preoperative radiation of head and neck cancer. Trans. Amer. Acad. Ophthal. Otolaryng. *72:* 937–942 (1968).
6. STRONG, B. W.; HENSCHKE, U. K.; NICKSON, J. J.; FRAZELL, B. L.; TOLLEFSEN, H. R., and HILARIS, B. S.: Preoperative X-Ray therapy as an adjunct to radical neck dissection. Cancer, Philad. *19:* 1,509–1,516 (1966).

Authors' address: Dr. HUGH F. BILLER and Dr. JOSEPH H. OGURA, Department of Otolaryngology, Washington University School of Medicine 517 S. Euclid, *St. Louis, MO 63110* (USA).

Front. Radiation Ther. Onc., vol. 5, pp. 106–122
(Karger, Basel/München/Paris/New York 1970)

Combined High Dose Radiation Therapy
and Surgery of Advanced Cancer
of the Laryngopharynx

S. M. SILVERSTONE[1], J. L. GOLDMAN, and J. R. RYAN

Departments of Radiotherapy and Oto-Laryngology, The Mount Sinai Hospital, New York,
N. Y.

Cancer of the larynx has always been the special domain for the radiotherapist because of the high cure rate of the early cases and their excellent functional results. One of the major reasons for this success is that the symptom of hoarseness alerts us to the possibility of cancer of the vocal cord and allows for its early detection. However, when this symptom goes unheeded or if the malignant neoplasm should arise in some other part of the larynx or laryngopharynx, then the growth can attain a large size before its presence is even suspected and by that time it could have reached an advanced stage with cervical lymph node metastasis. The results of treatment of advanced cancer of the laryngopharynx have been disappointingly poor by either radiation therapy or surgery as the sole method of treatment or even if surgery is employed for the radiation failures, or, vice versa, irradiation for surgical failures. It is to these advanced cases of laryngopharyngeal cancer that we have directed our efforts and our research program since 1958 to achieve a better cure rate.

Causes of Failure

There were three major causes of failure with either radiation therapy or surgery as the sole method of treatment: distant

---

[1] Clinical Professor of Radiotherapy, The Mount Sinai School of Medicine, New York, N. Y., Attending Radiotherapist, The Mount Sinai Hospital, New York, N. Y.

metastasis, regional lymph node metastasis, and local recurrence. A fourth cause of failure is a non-related fatal disease.

Distant Metastasis

Distant metastasis occurs late in the disease, usually several years after onset. While nothing curative is at present available, the fact that it does occur late in the natural history of laryngo-pharyngeal cancer is a further stimulus to attack this disease vigorously while it is yet localized to the region of the neck, no matter how extensive.

Regional Lymph Node Metastases

Metastases in the cervical lymph nodes are common, often the first clinical manifestation of the disease, in marked contrast to their rarity in the early vocal cord malignant lesions. Because of the frequency of their involvement, the cervical lymph nodes must be included in any plan of therapy. In the presence of metastatic cervical lymph nodes, there is a precipitous drop in the cure rate at any stage of development of the primary tumor.

Local Recurrence

After radiation therapy, local recurrence is probably the most common cause of failure. It is for this reason that the combined method of radiation therapy for the primary neoplasm and neck dissection for the metastatic cervical lymph nodes has not resulted in a better cure rate. The recurrent growth appears several months to a few years after radiation therapy is completed, often at the original site.

Its appearance is obscured at first by late radiation effects, particularly chronic interstitial edema and fibrosis. Biopsy is indicated but biopsy of an irradiated larynx is an unsatisfactory procedure. It involves a risk of ulceration at the biopsy site, while a negative report is not always reliable because the recurrent disease is often at a deeper submucosal level. When a positive biopsy is finally obtained, the recurrent disease may be as extensive as the original disease was before radiation therapy was instituted.

Repetition of radiation therapy is contra-indicated because of the risk of radionecrosis. Surgery would in all probability be performed if feasible, and some cases are salvaged, but the prognosis, nevertheless, is as poor as it was originally.

After radical surgery, local recurrence appears as prominent and palpable solid nodules within the operative site, often at the tracheostomy stoma. It may be the result of implantation of carcinoma cells during the surgical procedure, or the growth of tumor cell foci in the deeper fascial planes of the neck that technically were beyond the radical surgical excision. Recurrent nodules are rarely encapsuled masses that can be completely excised. They invariably infiltrate the surrounding tissues and their excision is too often promptly followed by further recurrence. Treatment therefore must be radiation therapy directed over a wide area. Unfortunately this therapy cannot always be applied effectively or adequately because the tissues comprising the tumor bed in the operative site are fibrotic and poorly vascularized. Therefore, radiation therapy for post-operative recurrence cannot be expected to add significantly to the cure rate.

Principles of Combined Therapy

The most significant observation in radiation therapy of advanced cancer of the laryngopharynx was the marked regression of the neoplasm at the completion of the course of therapy. Often there was no clinical evidence of neoplasm and the larynx had a normal or near normal appearance on indirect laryngoscopy. This favorable status continued for an unpredictable period. It could be weeks, months, or even years before recurrence set in. Then the patient quickly relapsed to the same unfavorable status he had before radiation therapy. We therefore reasoned that since the recurrence rate was so high that surgery had to be considered for most of the cases, the proper time for surgery should be during the early post irradiation period when the tumor was reduced to its minimum and the normal tissues comprising the tumor bed were in their best physiological state. To wait longer incurs not only the risk of an actively growing recurrent neoplasm but also the adverse effects of skin atrophy and telangiectasia, fibrosis, chronic interstitial edema, and endarteritis so characteristic of late radiation changes.

It was on the basis of this reasoning that we proposed to combine high dose radiation therapy with radical surgery in an integrated and strictly coordinated program. It must be stressed that this combined therapy program is not the same as operating for a radiation failure. Essentially, it is a unit method of treatment based upon radiobiological principles which we shall develop further in this discussion.

Combined Therapy Program

The combined therapy program is a joint enterprise of the laryngological surgeon and the radiotherapist, both of whom work together in all its active phases and in the follow-up studies. The program comprises three phases: (1) Preoperative irradiation with cobalt 60 teletherapy for a tumor dose of 5,500 R in 5 to 6 weeks, five fractions per week. (2) Post-radiation rest interval of 3 to 6 weeks. (3) Radical surgery.

Preoperative Irradiation

In the planning of the pre-operative irradiation, our first concern was to determine the volume of irradiation, that is, what tissues and structures must be irradiated. When that was determined, the problem arose as to dose, technique of administration, and quality of radiation to be employed. Finally there were the radiation reactions to be considered.

Volume of Irradiation

In addition to general medical evaluation, the preliminary work-up of every patient includes all clinical and roentgenological methods of study to determine the exact extent of the neoplasm.

Cancer of the laryngopharynx often involves contiguous structures such as the valleculae and base of tongue, the pre-epiglottic space, the lateral pharyngeal wall, and the trachea. All of these contiguous structures therefore are included in the volume of irradiation together with the entire laryngopharynx.

The extent of lymph node metastasis can be determined clinically only by palpation. Whether a palpable node is metastatic or inflammatory is a matter of clinical interpretation by the examiner. As a general rule, biopsy of cervical nodes is not done because the plan of combined therapy includes radical neck dissection on the involved side, or on both sides if indicated, whether the nodes are palpable or not. Unnecessary technical difficulties in the radical operation would be introduced if a node biopsy was done, while no particular advantage would be gained. Therefore, to include the entire laryngopharynx with its contiguous structures and the lymph node chains on both sides of the neck, the volume to be irradiated (fig. 1) must extend from the mandible and mastoid process to the junction of the neck with the shoulder, and from the coronal plane through the bodies of the cervical vertebrae to the anterior margin of the neck, including the submental triangle. Occasionally this volume may have to be enlarged further superiorly, posteriorly, or inferiorly because of more extensive lymph node involvement. Although the irradiation volume is as extensive and as inclusive of the tumor and all tumor bearing structures as the radical surgery that follows, it is actually greater in extent because it includes the skin and the deep fascia of the neck which are possible harborers of tumor foci but which cannot be included in the surgical excision.

If roentgenograms of the treatment fields show inclusion of the cervical spinal cord, some adjustment of the treatment field is desirable during the course of therapy so as not to exceed 3,500 R to the spinal cord segment of the irradiation volume and thus avoid the risk of radiation myelitis.

Dose of Irradiation

The response of squamous carcinoma cells to irradiation is dependent not only upon the intrinsic radiosensitivity of the cells but also upon their oxygenation and the character of the tumor bed. Blood supply, the infiltration of submucosa, connective tissue, muscle, cartilage or bone, and the size and bulkiness of the tumor also influence the radiation response. Consequently, in every advanced tumor, there is a wide spectrum of dosage response. Small nests of tumor cells in well vascularized tissues are easily destroyed by small doses of the order of 1,500 or 2,000 R

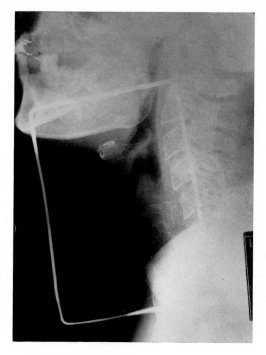

Fig. 1. Lateral roentgenogram of neck with outline of treatment field.

in 1½ to 2 weeks while bulky necrotic tumor masses infiltrating muscle or cartilage or bone may show only temporary mitotic inhibition with doses higher than 7,000 R at the same rate.

The objective of radiation therapy is to effect the maximum destruction and mitotic inhibition of cancer cells within the limits of tolerance of normal tissues, particularly those tissues and structures that will be subjected to radical surgery. On the basis of our radiation therapy experience, we determined that a tumor dose of 5,500 R administered over a 5-week period would be the maximum safe dose for the large volume of the neck that must be irradiated. This dose should destroy all of the rapidly growing, highly radiosensitive cancer foci, such as might be found in the peripheral areas of tumor growth. In the less sensitive and more radioresistant cell masses found in the bulkier tumors and in the muscle, cartilage, bone and fibrous tissue infiltrations, this dose should effect a prolonged period of mitotic inhibition. Furthermore, this dose is sufficiently well tolerated by the normal tissues so that the subsequent radical surgery can be successfully performed with minimal complications and with reasonable expectation of good wound healing.

Technique of Irradiation

The irradiation of this large volume of tissue is effected technically by parallel opposing lateral cervical fields. These treatment fields vary from 8 by 6 cm in a small neck to as much as 12 by 11 cm in larger necks, and in special circumstances, even larger. With this technique a good distribution of dosage is obtained. Roentgenograms are made with lead wire outline to record the volume that is being irradiated. The treatment volume is also recorded by a roentgenogram made with the actual beam of irradiation. The treatment field is outlined on the patient's neck with marking ink, such as carbol fuchsin, not only for reproducibility but also as a check on its adequacy, that all palpable nodes are included within it. Treatments are administered daily, alternately to each side, 5 times weekly over a 5- or 6-week period. They are generally so well tolerated that they can be given on an ambulatory basis.

Quality of Radiation

For a dose of 5,500 R in 5 weeks to this large neck region, radiation of supervoltage quality is essential. This implies the use of cobalt 60 teletherapy, 2 million volt x-ray machine, linear accelerator, or betatron. Cobalt 60 teletherapy is the most practical and it is the method we have employed.

It would be impossible to administer so high a dose with irradiation in the ortho-voltage range, 200 to 400 kV, because of the severe skin reactions and underlying fibrosis induced by that quality of radiation. The most valuable characteristic of supervoltage radiation is its skin sparing. The skin reaction at 5,500 R in 5 weeks is minimal, a light erythema followed by moderate pigmentation, slight scaling, and subsequent healing to a normal appearance with loss of hair.

Radiation Reactions

During the course of radiation therapy, the radiation reactions first appear about the 3rd week and continue to the end. They are minimal to moderate in intensity and are well tolerated. The principal clinical reactions are dryness of the pharyngeal mucosa with loss of taste, dysphagia, and hoarseness. Occasionally dysphagia is severe enough to necessitate lowering the daily tumor dose rate and thereby prolonging the overall treatment time to about 6 weeks instead of 5 as originally planned. Tumor regression associated with fibrinous membrane formation is best followed by mirror laryngoscopy. The response of lymph nodes is less constant and more variable. Large nodes become smaller, fixed nodes become movable, some nodes may disappear. Occasionally a bulky metastatic node mass may show no change in size clinically but on subsequent surgery this mass is found to be cystic and it may have no viable cells in its fluid contents.

Post-Irradiation Rest Interval

At about three weeks after completion of the radiation therapy, the reactions have subsided. Regression of the primary neoplasm and the involved cervical nodes has probably reached its maximum while residual tumor is in a state of mitotic inhibition. At this time the patient looks well and has improved his nutritional status. His laryngopharynx and his neck are in their best physiological status, the best they ever will be. On indirect laryngoscopy, the larynx may have a normal appearance. At this favorable stage it is sometimes difficult to persuade a patient to undergo the necessary radical surgery. However our knowledge of the ultimate fatal prognosis of these cases must prevail. This rest interval should not exceed 6 weeks. No further advantages are gained, while a longer delay incurs the double risk of local recurrence and adverse late radiation changes in the normal tissues. The 3- to 6-week limitation of this rest interval is one of the basic and most important principles of our combined therapy program.

Radical Surgery

The surgery comprises wide-field laryngectomy and radical neck dissection with hemi-thyroidectomy. If bilateral neck dissection is indicated, the side with clinically greater involvement is done first. The second side should be done as soon as feasible, generally within a few weeks. The extent of the surgery must be as planned originally, before the onset of the radiation therapy. The principle of the surgical phase is that the operation should be as radical as it would have been if no radiation therapy had been given. The purpose of the radiation therapy is not to reduce the surgery but to make it more effective and to eliminate the risk of local recurrence.

Complications

In most cases wound healing has been good. There have probably been more postoperative complications than usual because of the radiation effects. The more frequent complications were wound infections, fistulas, and skin necrosis, some of which required plastic surgery. Less frequent complications included stricture, chyle leak, exposure of the carotid artery, and one case of hemorrhage.

These complications have been reduced by several surgical measures developed during our experience with combined therapy. Preoperatively the skin of the operative area is prepared for one week with twice daily phisohex scrubs. A modified apron flap has been devised which gives excellent exposure of the operative site, provides protection for the carotid artery, and, in addition, gives a good cosmetic result. At the time of the surgery, hemostasis is meticulous and large arteries, such as the superior thyroid and carotid, are protected by muscle flaps. The pharynx is closed in three layers to prevent fistula. Intermittent suction drainage is used to maintain flap coaptation and prevent hematoma. A soft rubber drain at the posterior-inferior margin of the apron flap is directed toward the pharyngeal suture line. Postoperatively, autibiotics are given prophylactically. Naso-gastric feedings, started on the second postoperative day, are continued for two weeks before the patient is allowed to swallow food. All these technical measures have reduced complications to an acceptable level.

Every case thus far has healed completely. The tracheostomy functions well without a tube. There is minimal muscle disability in the neck even with bilateral neck dissection. Most patients have learned a useful esophageal voice.

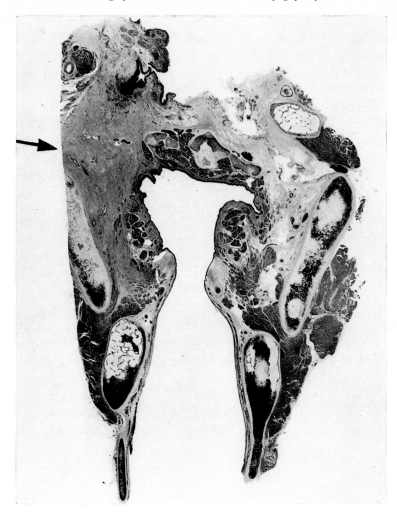

Fig. 2. Whole larynx section showing minute residual nest of tumor cells in deeper tissues.

Histopathology of the Larynx

The routine histological method of examining the surgically excised larynx lacks the thoroughness necessary in the search for residual cancer. A special histological project was therefore undertaken in which the surgically excised larynx was preserved in toto as a unit, fixed and processed until it was embedded in celloidin. Serial sections of the whole larynx were then made in the coronal plane (fig. 2). With this more thorough method of study, residual cancer was found histologically in cases that clinically, on mirror laryngoscopy, appeared to be free of disease. The reverse was also true. In two cases that appeared to be clinically positive, residual cancer could not be found histologically. This lack of correlation between the clinical and the histological findings clearly indicates that clinical evaluation of an irradiated larynx by mirror laryngoscopy is not a reliable method of determining the presence or absence of residual cancer.

A histological observation of major importance is that the residual tumor was found in the form of tumor cell nests, 0.5 to 1.8 mm in diameter, rarely larger. Furthermore, these cell nests were randomly scattered in the submucosa at some distance in depth from the completely intact mucous membrane over them (fig. 3). They could not possibly have been seen or even suspected on examination by mirror laryngoscopy, and even biopsy could easily miss them.

During radiation therapy the reduction in size of the tumor is often observed to be centripetal in character, that is, the periphery of the tumor is the first area to disappear while the central portion, presumed to be the site of origin, is the last. If this observation is entirely correct then the postradiation surgery could be less extensive. However, the histological finding of minute cell nests scattered in depth invalidates this clinical observation. Our original premise that surgery must be extensive and cannot be modified still holds in the light of these histological findings.

Histopathology of the Lymph Nodes

The routine histological examination of the lymph nodes is at best incomplete and inadequate because of the enormous amount of work involved if the entire operative specimen were to be minutely examined. Therefore the radical neck dissection specimens were processed *in toto*, like the larynges, in a celloidin block and cut serially. With this more thorough method of histological examination, microscopic cancer was found in nodes which were not

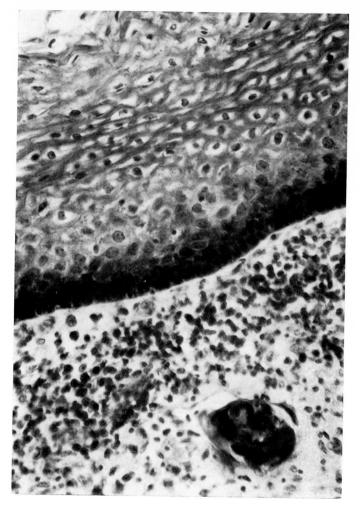

Fig. 3. Residual nest of tumor cells covered by intact mucous membrane.

palpable before operation. However considerable destruction of cancer cells was also demonstrated, thus confirming the clinical observation that lymph node metastasis can be destroyed by irradiation.

One observation of special practical importance is that tumor cells were found only in lymph nodes. No tumor cells were found in tissues outside a lymph node. The deduction from this observation is that preoperative irradiation destroys cancer cells lying freely in the connective tissues, cells which could otherwise have been a potential source of local recurrence after surgery.

Mitotic Inhibition

The concept of mitotic inhibition resulting from radiation therapy is inferred clinically by the long delay in the appearance of a local recurrence in those cases treated only by irradiation. This delay is measured in months or years. When re-growth does take place, the cancer cells manifest the same growth potential and growth rate that the original tumor had before irradiation. With the appearance of this new generation of cancer cells the effectiveness of the previous radiation therapy is completely nullified. Instead there exists a neoplasm growing rapidly in tissues partially devitalized and more vulnerable to trauma and infection. The patient has relapsed to his original unfavorable pre-radiation status.

It is difficult if not impossible to ascertain on histological examination which cells were viable in the post-radiation nests of tumor cells, that is, viable to the extent of eventually reproducing themselves as cancer cells after the mitotic inhibitory effect of the radiation had worn off. That such cells exist we infer from the very fact of recurrence itself.

Viability has recently been studied with tritium labelled thymidine, a nucleoside which is incorporated into DNA molecules during the DNA synthesis phase which precedes mitosis by several hours. By radioautographs, the amount of DNA activity can be inferred by the number of silver granules precipitated out of the silver photographic emulsion by the beta particles emitted by the radioactive tritium. Biopsy specimens taken before and during the course of radiation therapy and incubated with tritium labelled thymidine showed, by this technique, that there was not only a marked reduction in the number of tritium labelled tumor cells but also a reduction in the amount of DNA activity in the cells so labelled. It was significant that even after 5,500 R some cells were synthesizing DNA. This finding could be interpreted as evidence of viability.

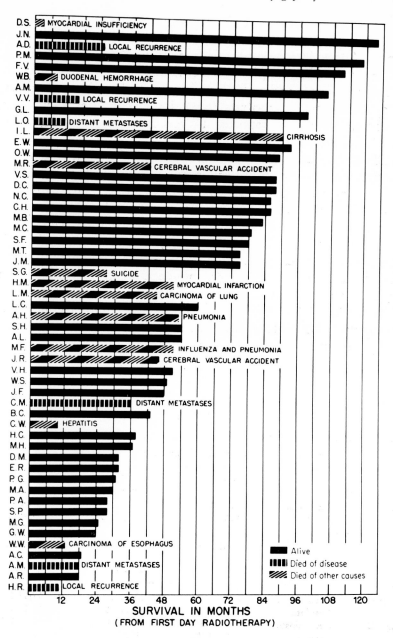

Fig. 4. Patient survival.

Clinical Results

From 1958 to 1969, 53 cases of advanced squamous cell carcinoma of the laryngopharynx (fig. 4) were treated by combined high-dose radiation therapy and radical surgery and 35 are alive and well today. The detailed analysis (table I) of staging and cure rates has been adequately reported in recent publications and need only be summarized here.

Of the 18 deaths (table II) that occurred during this period of study, 3 were due to local recurrence, 3 to distant metastases, and 12 to other non-related fatal diseases. In none of the latter was there evidence of local recurrence at the time of death.

In addition to the 3 cases of local recurrence, there were 2 cases of contralateral lymph node recurrence, none ipsilateral (table III). Thus only 5 cases were direct failures of combined therapy. Combined therapy can have no influence on the development of distant metastases or a non-related fatal disease. Therefore, in 48 cases out of 53, combined therapy successfully accomplished its objective, which is to eradicate locally advanced cancer of the laryngopharynx, a local cure rate of 90%.

Table I. Survival rates

		International classification					
		5-Year		3-Year		2-Year	
Stage III	Determinate	18/21	86%	33/36	92%	44/46	96%
	Absolute	18/27	67%	33/40	83%	44/49	90%
		American classification					
		5-Year		3-Year		2-Year	
Stage II	Determinate	2/2	100%	10/10	100%	17/17	100%
	Absolute	2/5	40%	10/11	91%	17/17	100%
Stage III	Determinate	4/5	80%	8/9	89%	9/9	100%
	Absolute	4/7	57%	8/10	80%	9/10	90%
Stage IV	Determinate	12/14	86%	15/17	88%	18/20	90%
	Absolute	12/15	80%	15/19	79%	18/22	82%

Table II

Total cases		53
Survivals		35
Dead of disease		6
Local recurrence	3	
Distant metastases	3	
Dead of other causes		12

Table III. Local effectiveness of combined therapy

Total number of cases		53
Failures of local eradication		5
Local recurrence	3	
Ipsilateral cervical recurrence	0	
Contralateral cervical recurrence	2	
Successful local eradication		48 (90%)

Summary and Conclusions

1. Locally advanced squamous cell carcinoma of the laryngopharynx with cervical lymph node metastasis can be eradicated by preoperative irradiation for a dose of 5,500 R in 5 to 6 weeks followed in 3 to 6 weeks by radical surgery.

2. Both irradiation and surgery are well tolerated. Wound healing has been good and complications have been reduced by special surgical details.

3. The irradiation destroys most of the primary tumor and reduces the residuum to nests of cells in a temporary state of mitotic inhibition, scattered randomly in the deeper tissues and generally unrecognizable on mirror laryngoscopy.

4. Metastatic lymph nodes are also reduced, some are destroyed. Fixed nodes become mobile. Extranodal tumor cells are destroyed and residual tumor foci remain within the lymph node.

5. The irradiation must be directed to all the tumor bearing structures of the neck which are then totally excised during the post-radiation phase of mitotic inhibition.

6. Combined therapy has been effective in eradicating the locally advanced laryngopharyngeal cancer in 90% of our cases.

References

1. American Joint Committee: Clinical staging system for cancer of the larynx (June 1962).
2. FLETCHER, G. H. and JESSE, R. H., Jr.: Contribution of supervoltage roentgenotherapy to integration of radiation and surgery in head and neck squamous cell carcinomas. Cancer *15:* 566–577 (1962).
3. FRIEDMAN, W. H. and GOLDMAN, J. L.: Tritiated thymidine studies of radiated laryngeal cancer. Arch. Otolaryng. *89:* 766–769 (1969).
4. GOLDMAN, J. L.; BLOOM, B. S.; ZAK, F. G.; FRIEDMAN, W. H.; GUNSBERG, M. J., and SILVERSTONE, S. M.: Serial microscopic studies of radical neck dissections. Arch. Otolaryng. *89:* 620–628 (1969).
5. GOLDMAN, J. L.; CHEREN, R. V.; ZAK, F. G., and GUNSBERG, M. J.: Histopathology of larynges and radical neck specimens in a combined radiation and surgery program for advanced carcinoma of the larynx and laryngopharynx. Ann. Otol. Rhinol. Laryng. *75:* 313–335 (1966).
6. GOLDMAN, J. L. and FRIEDMAN, W. H.: The intranuclear tracer, cell viability and preoperative irradiation. Laryngoscope *77:* 1315–1327 (1967).
7. GOLDMAN, J. L.; FRIEDMAN, W. H., and BLOOM, B. S.: Elective neck dissection in laryngeal and laryngopharyngeal cancer. Laryngoscope *78:* 539–548 (1968).
8. GOLDMAN, J. L. and SILVERSTONE, S. M.: The role of radiation therapy in carcinoma of the larynx. Ann. Otol. Rhinol. Laryng. *69:* 890–895 (1960).
9. GOLDMAN, J. L.; SILVERSTONE, S. M.; ROSIN, H. D.; CHEREN, R. V., and ZAK, F. G.: Combined radiation and surgical therapy for cancer of the larynx and laryngopharynx II. Laryngoscope *74:* 1,111–1,134 (1964).
10. HARRIS, W.; SILVERSTONE, S. M., and KRAMER, R.: Roentgen therapy for cancer of larynx and laryngopharynx. Amer. J. Roentgenol. *71:* 813–825 (1954).
11. HENSCHKE, U. K.; FRAZELL, E. L.; HILARIS, B. S.; NICKSON, J. J.; TOLLEFSEN, H. R., and STRONG, E. W.: Local recurrences after radical neck dissection with and without preoperative X-ray therapy. Radiology *82:* 331–332 (1964). Value of preoperative X-ray therapy as an adjunct to radical neck dissection. Radiology *86:* 450–453 (1966).
12. REED, G. F.: Preoperative irradiation in laryngeal carcinoma. Arch. Otolaryng. *86:* 318–325 (1967).
13. ROXO-NOBRE, M. O.: Clinical stage classification of malignant tumors of larynx. Acta Un. int. Cancer *16:* 1,865–1,873 (1960).
14. SILVERSTONE, S. M.; GOLDMAN, J. L., and ROSIN, H. D.: Combined therapy, irradiation and surgery, for advanced cancer of the laryngopharynx. Amer. J. Roentgenol. *90:* 1,023–1,031 (1963).
15. SILVERSTONE, S. M. and SIMON, N.: Advantages of cobalt-60 in practice of radiotherapy. J. Mt Sinai Hosp. *24:* 124–136 (1957).

Author's address: Dr. SIDNEY M. SILVERSTONE, 945 Fifth Avenue, *New York, NY 10021* (USA).

Front. Radiation Ther. Onc., vol. 5, pp. 123–129
(Karger, Basel/München/Paris/New York 1970)

The Results of Low Dose
Preoperative Radiotherapy for Advanced
Carcinoma of the Larynx

F. R. HENDRICKSON

University of Illinois and Section of Radiation Therapy, Presbyterian-St. Luke's Hospital
Chicago, Ill.

The principles upon which the rational basis of preoperative radiotherapy are founded have been well expounded in the literature [1–4] and have been enumerated by other authors in this volume. These studies include both treatment of experimental tumors in animals, as well as a number of clinical investigations. The consensus from this work would suggest that the growing perimeter of a tumor is sufficiently injured by less than curative doses of radiation to reduce the incidence of local regrowth after surgical removal. Whether this is a function of better oxygenation, a different cell cycle time, a larger proportion of non-viable cells, or even a local affect on the tumor bed may be of intense interest, but not relevant to the clinical application of the observed effect.

In 1963 a combined project between the radiation therapy departments of the University of Illinois Research and Education Hospital, and the Presbyterian-St. Luke's Hospital was undertaken to investigate the feasibility and effects of preoperative radiotherapy for advanced laryngeal carcinomas. The reasons for choosing carcinoma of the larynx as a suitable test site were:

1. In order to test effectiveness of combined treatment, tumors with predominantly local failure are most suitable. As discussed in previous papers, patients with tumors such as carcinoma of the lung and breast die predominantly from distant metastases which greatly obscures the combined treatment effect on local control of disease.

2. The two institutions have a large referral of laryngeal lesions seeing jointly nearly 100 new cases a year of which roughly one-fourth are suitable for such combined treatment.

From 1963 to 1965 a random assignment to radiation dose levels of either 2000 R in 2 weeks or 5000 R in 4 weeks was made on the basis of birthdate. Preliminary analysis of this trial prompted a revision in 1967 to include in random assignment to surgery only and elimination of the higher dose group. Additional institutions have joined this prospective study, however the follow up duration is insufficient at this time to comment on salvage results. Over 260 patients with advanced lesions of the larynx have now been treated with preoperative radiotherapy. Although all of these patients are treated under the same protocol, only those patients from our institutions are presented here.

Specifics of Treatment

The radiotherapy protocol specified that all preoperative radiotherapy be given with super-voltage equipment. The treatment fields were arranged to include all of the primary tumor, and clinical palpable adenopathy if such were present, or the most likely involved regional nodes for other patients. In general, field sizes varied from a minimum of 6×10 cm to 8×15 cm. In the dose level comparison portion of the study daily tumor doses were always 250 R with total doses of 2,000 R in 8 treatments, or 5,000 R in 20 treatments. Depending on conversion factors for the NSD the lower dose represents about two-thirds of tolerance and the higher dose in excess of 90% of tolerance dose levels. During the more recent portion of the study, patients have been randomized to receive: (1) surgery only, (2) a two dose pre-operative treatment with 650 to 700 R delivered at each of two fractions separated 48 to 96 hours, (3) 2,000 R delivered in 8 treatments over 10 days. These 2 preoperative dose levels seem nearly equivalent in biologic effectiveness and were chosen to investigate the simplest logistics for preoperative treatment. Because of the factor of tumor cell anoxia and reoxygena-tion it was felt that single dose preoperative treatment was not advisable and with the higher increment doses that probably a longer fraction interval would be appropriate.

In all cases the surgical procedure consisted of a standard laryngectomy and almost always a radical neck dissection on the involved side. Occasionally for patients with midline lesions and no demonstrable adenopathy laryngectomy only was the surgery performed. After low dose treatment surgery is performed promptly. After the higher dose, surgery is delayed 4 to 6 weeks to permit the acute reaction to heal.

Results

In investigating the interval at which results can be reasonably assessed one must look to the rate of recurrence or failure. A review of our own material would indicate that some 90% of local tumor failure has occurred by 24 months. This would be in keeping with published results of others for squamous cell lesions in the head and neck area. [5] This, of course, does not mean that additional failures do not occur later in time, however, the failure from intercurrent disease or other primary tumors plays a significant role in the longer term survival. More than 10% of our patients failing to reach the 5-year level have failed to reach this level for reasons other than their laryngeal tumors. For this reason we have felt it reasonable to make a preliminary examination of the results at the 2-year level. Table I compares the 2-year tumor free survival for patients in the 2,000 versus the 5,000 R dose. Stage by stage comparison of patients treated at each institution showed no significance in variation so they are combined for presentation. At this time it was evident that the higher dose level was no more effective in the operable patients. The lack of a surgery only control was glaring and the randomization technique was not yielding even distribution of patients. The second study was therefore undertaken, although patients accrued into the first study were continually followed. Table II indicates the 4-year results for essentially the same group except patients not operated upon are excluded and a few additional patients are available for analysis. Although the results from the random assignment to surgery only are not yet matured, an effort to assess the surgery only results has been made by reviewing the patients treated at our institutions from 1961 to 1963. These results are presented in table III. Assessment either by T or by N would suggest that the preoperative group may be doing somewhat better.

Table I. Staging and 2-year tumor free results of supraglottic primary squamous cell carcinoma assigned to random study from June, 1963 to June, 1965

	2,000 R dose				5,000 R dose			
	T2	T3	T4	Total	T2	T3	T4	Total
N0	2/3	7/10	1/2	10/15	2/2	8/13[1]	3/6[1]	13/21
N1	1/1	2/3[1]	0/0	3/4	1/2	4/4	3/4	8/10
N2	1/3[1]	0/2	0/1	1/6	0/0	0/2[1]	0/1	0/3
Total	4/7	9/15	1/3	14/25	3/4	12/19	6/11	21/34

[1] Indicates number and location of patients admitted to the study but on whom surgery was never performed but still carried in the series as a failure.

Table II. Carcinoma of the larynx preoperative radiation therapy 4 years NED survival 2,000 rads vs. 5,000 rads

	2,000 rads				
	T1	T2	T3	T4	Total
N0		4/4	7/13	0/1	11/18
N1		1/1	4/5		5/6
N2	1/1	0/1	0/2	0/1	1/5
Total	1/1	5/6	11/20	0/2	17/29 (58%)

	5,000 rads				
	T1	T2	T3	T4	Total
N0		0/4	7/10	4/6	11/20
N1	0/1	5/6	4/5	0/7	9/19
N2			1/3		1/3
Total	0/1	5/10	12/18	4/13	21/42 (50%)

[1] Note 6 patients died of intercurrent disease before the 4th year without evidence of recurrent or metastatic larynx cancer.

Table III. Two-year tumor–free survival of supraglottic primary squamous cell carcinoma completing surgery

	T2	T3	T4	Total
Surgery only 1961–1963	7/14 (50%)	4/8 (50%)	1/6 (17%)	12/28 (43%)
Preoperative irrad. 1963–1965	7/10 (70%)	21/30 (70%)	7/13 (54%)	35/53 (66%)
	N0	N1	N2	Total
Surgery only 1961–1963	9/16 (56%)	3/9 (33%)	0/3 (0)	12/28 (43%)
Preoperative irrad.	23/33 (70%)	11/13 (85%)	1/7 (14%)	35/53 (66%)

Table IV. Comparison of complication rates

	Fistulae	Wound infection	Deaths	Averaged estimated blood-loss
Preoperative group				
5,000 rads	7/36	6/36	2/36	1,280 ml
2,000 rads	2/16	2/12	0/12	1,340 ml
No preoperative therapy				
Laryngo-pharynx	6/42	3/42	1/46	1,270 ml
Tongue	0/12	3/12	0/12	

Considerable concern was initially expressed about the complications of combined treatment. Because of this concern it should be emphasized that meticulous surgical technique has been maintained. Excellent hemostasis has been secured and the flaps have been drained wherever indicated for a moderate length of time. When feeding tubes have been required, they have been left in a day or two longer than usual. While fistula formation has still been a problem, major wound infection and flap breakdown has not been an unduly frequent complication. Table IV compares the complications in the preoperative group with a similar group of patients undergoing comparable kinds of surgery. While the end results of the cooperative multi-institution clinical trial are not reportable as yet it can be stated that the complications rate has been no different in the surgery only and in the preoperative group for the first one hundred patients.

The overall survival of the 104 patients from our institution is presented in figure 1. The 91 patients assessable at the 2-year interval are broken down into detailed fashion in table V, the overall results have the trends anticipated. The T2 lesions were predominantly large supraglottic tumors but did not extend into the glottis. One of these measured 4 cm in the excised larynx. As reported previously [2] half of the N_0 patients had microscopic tumor in the neck specimen. It is particularly significant that the patients with fixed nodal disease in the neck have minimal benefit possibly indicating that such fixed disease is not truly operable, and should not be considered for a low dose preoperative program. Possibly a higher dose of irradiation combined with surgery or irradiation alone or combined with chemotherapy would be more suitable.

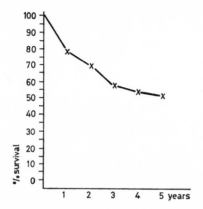

Fig. 1. The survival curve is based upon 104 patients at 1 year, 91 patients at 2 years to 54 patients at 5 years.

Table V. Carcinoma of larynx preoperative radiation therapy 2 year NED

	T1	T2	T3	T4	Total
N0		8/12	25/33 (75%)	9/10	42/55 (76%)
N1		4/5	7/8	5/9	16/22 (73%)
N2	1/1	0/2	1/7	1/4	3/14
Total	1/1	12/19	33/48 (68%)	15/23	61/91 (67%)

Conclusions

At this time our feeling would be that, (1) for truly operable lesions low dose preoperative radiotherapy is equally as effective as high dose preoperative radiotherapy in improving survival. This technique has many advantages from the logistical point of view. (2) From limited experience with lesions which are inoperable, because of local extension, high dose preoperative therapy may occasionally convert such lesions to be technically operable and truly salvagable. However here the intent is to sterilize a tumor margin in tissue which must be left behind. (3) If one uses good surgical technique, judgement and general supportive care the complication rate from combined treatment seems to be no greater than from a comparably extensive procedure alone.

References

1. FEDER, B. H.; BLAIR, P. B., and CLOSE, P.: Fractionation in pre-operative irradiation. Radiology 84: 447–451 (1965).
2. HENDRICKSON, F. R. and LIEBNER, E.: Results of pre-operative radiotherapy for supra-glottic larynx cancer. Ann. Otol. Rhinol. Laryng. 77: 222 (1968).
3. NICKSON, J. J. and GLICKSMAN, A. S.: Pre-operative radiotherapy in cancer. J. amer. med. Ass. 195: 138–142 (1966).
4. POWERS, W. E.: Radiation biologic considerations and practical investigations in pre-operative radiation therapy. J. canad. Ass. Radiol. 16: 217–225 (1965).
5. SUIT, H.; WETTE, R., and LINDBERG, R.: Analysis of tumor-recurrence times. Radiology 88: 311–321 (1967).

Author's address: Prof. FRANK R. HENDRICKSON, Section of Radiation Therapy, Presbyterian-St. Luke's Hospital, Chicago, IL (USA).

Front. Radiation Ther. Onc., vol. 5, pp. 130–146
(Karger, Basel/München/Paris/New York 1970)

Carcinoma of the Paranasal Sinuses, Combined Approach

C.-A. HAMBERGER and G. MÅRTENSSON

Department of Otolaryngology and Department of Oral and Jaw Diseases, Karolinska
Sjukhuset, Stockholm

The most extensive presentation of the paranasal sinus tumors is found in a thesis from the Department of Otolaryngology in Stockholm by GEORG ÖHNGREN in 1933 [5]. He had the great privilege of close cooperation with the Radiumhemmet in Stockholm, and particularly with Professor ELIS BERVEN, at that time the chief of the clinic. From the very beginning conventional roentgen treatment was given, but later radiations of higher energy have gradually been introduced.

Before discussing our present experience of pre- and postoperative radiotherapy in the treatment we would like to say some words of a more common interest.

The Sensitivity of the Normal Tissue to Radiation

When radiotherapy is used for diseases in the nasal cavities and the paranasal sinuses, the skin, the bone structure and the cartilage in the skeleton of the face and the conchae as well as the mucous membrane in the nasal cavities are irradiated. The chronical changes of the skin caused by the radiation are confined to persisting epilation and slight atrophy. The bone tissues in the paranasal sinuses may sometimes, particularly after high radiation exposures, roentgenologically show a considerable loss of calcium but real bone necrosis is unusual and, for example, considerably more rare than radionecrosis of the mandible. Radiotherapy in the acute phase results in epithelité later on followed by mucous membrane atrophy.

The most pronounced technical inconvenience of radiotherapy in the region of the head is the sensitivity of the eye to ionizing radiation. Cataract can be obtained after exposures of 500 to 1,000 R; after still higher exposures panophthalmia and total destruction of the eye may occur. A large number of the tumors in this region are located in the proximity of the orbit, frequently causing destruction of the bone tissues of the orbit. Adequate protection of the eye from irradiation is then extremely difficult to accomplish and, sometimes, insuperable. It is therefore of essential importance to protect the eye on the healthy side almost entirely from irradiation. As concerns the eye on the tumor side, the course of procedure depends on the location of the tumor. If the tumor does not infiltrate the orbit or its walls, it is probably possible to protect the eye from direct irradiation. However, a certain amount of secondary radiation to the eye cannot be avoided, and even this can be high enough to produce a cataract. If the tumor infiltrates the orbit, the eye on this side may under all circumstances be considered as lost, if a curative treatment is strived for. Therefore, at the planning of the radiotherapy (as well as at the surgical treatment) a wish to preserve the eye should not hazard the aim at a curative treatment.

Malignant Tumors within the System of the Paranasal Sinuses

The malignant tumors can be grouped according to their radio-sensitivity.

1. *High radiosensitivity*. The tumor disappears practically always within the irradiated volume after relatively moderate exposures, 3,000 to 5,000 R in four weeks. Plasmocyte sarcoma, reticulum cell sarcoma and lymphosarcoma belong to this group.

2. *Moderate radiosensitivity*. Radiation exposures of 5,000 to 7,000 R in 6 weeks are here needed for a curative treatment, but even with exposures of this size it is, by no means, not always as sure that the tumor tissue completely disappears. The majority of the carcinomas, that is the majority of malignant tumors in this region, belong to this group. The radiosensitivity of the carcinomas seems, however, not to be constant. The anaplastic cancers are

most often highly radiosensitive, next the differentiated squamous
cell carcinomas, and last the cylindrical cell carcinomas.

3. *Low radiosensitivity.* Curative result in this group can, probably, only exceptionally be obtained by radiological methods.
However, radiotherapy can be justified in combination with
surgical treatment, and for palliative purpose. The mucous
secreting adenocarcinoma of the ethmoid, the malignant melanoma
as well as the mucous and the salivary gland tumors belong to this
group.

Treatment Principles

The reported scheme of different radiosensitivities gives a guidance
for the principles of treatment. The most suitable treatment in the
first group of highly radiosensitive tumors is radiotherapy, and
in the second group combined radiologic-surgical therapy. The
following presentation deals with group 2, that is the cancers
constituting the most dominating type of tumor in this region.
The principles of treatment are, however, more or less different
at various clinics, particularly in the operable cases. At certain
clinics they are only surgically treated, while at others surgical
treatment is combined with pre- or postoperative radiotherapy.
On the other hand many clinics prefer radiotherapy alone, even for
safely operable cases. At the Radiumhemmet preoperative external
radiotherapy is usually given, and about 6 weeks after the end of
the radiotherapy a radical operation is performed. Previously this
was often combined with local application of gamma radiation
sources inserted into the operation cavity.

Technique of External Radiotherapy

Roentgen therapy with radiation of maximum 200 kV energy
was earlier the only available technique. By cross fire irradiation,
or moving beam technique, a radiation exposure distribution as
favourable as possible was strived for.

This method, which during a long period has been used at
the Radiumhemmet, can be described as an example of such a
technique. The treatment was given by four rectangular facial

fields, two medial and two lateral, always directing the beam towards the center of the tumor. In permuted order one field is daily given a skin exposure of 400 to 500 R. Smaller daily exposures are given from the beginning, if the tumor is strongly infected, and the general state of the patient impaired. In the inoperable cases the prescribed skin exposure usually goes up to about 3,000 R to each field, which gives a total tumor exposure in the facial cavity of about 6,000 to 7,000 R in 30 to 35 days elapsed time. In the operable cases such an exposure is usually given preoperatively. The postoperative radiotherapy is then dispensed with. In some cases a rather small preoperative exposure is given, and the operation is then combined with radium inserted in the cavity. Before the beginning of the radiotherapy a Caldwell-Luc operation is performed to get both a histologic verification and a safe knowledge of the extension of the tumor and of its operability. At this operation a great part of the lateral wall of the maxillary sinus is removed to get an open communication into the oral cavity for inspection and drainage during the radio- therapy. Provided that the orbit on the tumor side has not been infiltrated, the eyes are shielded by lead during the irradia- tion. If infiltrated, the orbit at the tumor side should not be shielded from irradiation, or only be shielded during a part of the treatment.

Roentgen therapy with 200 kV radiation has, however, con- siderable disadvantages. Particularly in the treatment of tumors where the entire tumor region cannot safely be covered by each beam, the exposure distribution becomes very heterogeneous and, in certain parts of the tumor, the exposure will be considerably lower than desirable. Consequently, in more deep-seated tumors, it is not possible to attain a satisfactory radiation exposure. The considerable amount of bone tissue in this region will also con- tribute to reduce the depth exposure to a lower level than that calculated from homogeneous phantoms, and besides increases the energy absorbed in the bone tissues.

Radiotherapy was therefore very much improved by the intro- duction of new radioactive kilocurie sources, such as ^{60}Co, and new units for the production of alternatively high-energy roentgen radiation and electron beams. Linear accelerators and betatrons are well-known examples of such units, providing an almost ideal beam geometry due to an extremely small focus size, and radiations of much higher energy.

These new high-energy radiation sources have consequently attracted much interest in radiotherapy, particularly since an important skin-sparing effect as a function of the built-up depth, a strongly reduced absorption of energy in bone tissues as compared with that in soft tissues, and a considerable increase of the percentage depth doses were evident. All these characteristics have, in fact, proved to be of great clinical value.

As a rule, when high-energy radiation is used, it is possible to get an adequate distribution of the radiation exposure, for instance, by using a 2 or 3-field technique, or a moving beam technique. The use of wedge-filters is frequently suitable to avoid an over-exposure of certain parts of the irradiated volume, and in many cases this technique, using two fields on the tumor side, will be sufficient. The use of electron beams of 15–40 MeV has also been initiated. The sharply defined beams and the small amounts of scattered radiation account for a better protection of the normal tissues surrounding the irradiated volume, particularly of those behind the tumor region when electron beams are used.

Local Applications of Gamma Radiation Sources

Various techniques have been used for the application of gamma radiation sources in the maxillary sinus or the operation cavity. The radioactive source material was earlier radium, but during the later years even ^{60}Co or ^{137}Cs have been introduced. Insertion of long radioactive needles into the entire tumor field has also been used. Experiments with implantation of needles with radioactive iridium are under way. The advantage of those methods are that locally very high exposures can be obtained. The disadvantage is that the exposure, according to the inverse square law, is rapidly decreasing. There is thus considerable risk that the periphery of the tumor region, which in practice can be difficult to determine, will get too low an exposure.

At the Radiumhemmet radium applications have only been used in direct connection with operation. Four radium tubes of 50 mg each have been inserted into that part of the operative cavity where the security margin of radical treatment was smallest, that is usually the upper posterior part of the operative cavity. The exposure time was 3 to 5 hours depending on the size of the pre-operative radiation exposure.

At certain clinics radium application is the only radiologic treatment used. To get as great a deep-effect and as regularly distributed an exposure as possible, it has been attempted to center the radium containers in the maxillary sinus, or in the operative cavity, and to refer the exposure to a certain distance from the container, for instance to the surface of a sphere with a radius of 2 to 2.5 cm and with its center positioned in the container.

Using modern methods for external megavolt radiotherapy, however, the importance of the local, usually postoperative application methods is much reduced.

Results

Results from different clinics are difficult to compare due to the different composition of the patient material. Our material which partly has been described elsewhere [1, 2, 3, 4, 5], is the 5-year result from the period 1940 to 1964 at the Department of Oto-laryngology, Karolinska Sjukhuset. It comprises combined radio-logic and surgical treatment of operable cases, and only radiologic treatment of mainly inoperable cases. The surgical treatment was carried out at the Department of Otolaryngology.

Definition of the Series

The investigation was confined to carcinomas of the mucous membranes of the paranasal sinuses and the nasal cavities. Although this limitation is logical from the anatomic point of view, it may present some difficulties in practice. Particularly tumors from the maxillary gingiva may show secondary growth into the nasal cavity or the paranasal sinuses and may be difficult to distinguish from true nasosinusal tumors. It is nevertheless our opinion that, in the majority of cases, a careful study of the history and of the

clinical and roentgenologic findings will enable a determination
of the primary site with a high degree of probability. In a few
advanced cases such a limitation was not possible, but they are
nevertheless included in the series.

With regard to histologic type the investigation was confined
to carcinoma, which is the most common malignant tumor of
this region. Malignant tumors of the mucous and salivary glands
were excluded.

Composition of the Series

From 1940 to 1964 inclusive, a total of 648 patients with carcinoma
arising from the paranasal sinuses or the nasal cavities were
referred to our Department. However, 81 of them were not
admitted. This latter group consisted of patients in whom any
form of therapy was considered useless, due to advanced age or
poor general state.

The age distribution shows that these tumors are very
rare in ages up to 30 years, and relatively uncommon before
the age of 40. The youngest patient was a 19-year-old woman
(fig. 1).

All experience shows that carcinoma in this region mostly
arises from the mucous membranes of the maxillary or the ethmoid
sinus, the former showing an evident dominance. In view of the
intimate relation between the paranasal sinuses, it is often impossible to determine the primary site. Primary carcinomas of the
frontal and the sphenoid sinus are very uncommon. In fact, the
series included only one case with a primary localization to the
former sinus and none to the latter.

Histologic Examination

It is important to realize that the early symptoms and signs are
unspecific, and that a roentgen film 'without signs of bone
destruction' never excludes a malignant tumor. Chronic sinusitis
should not be treated conservatively for a long period, and when
tissue is removed at minor operations (removal of polyps,
Caldwell-Luc operation), specimens should be sent for histologic

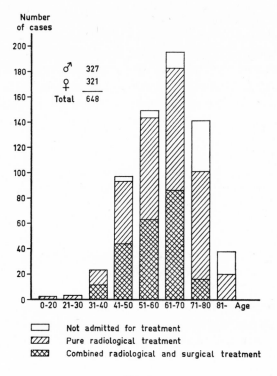

Fig. 1

Table I. Histopathologic diagnosis

Squamous cell carcinoma, well-differentiated	250
Squamous cell carcinoma, poorly differentiated	101
Cylindric cell carcinoma	54
Cylindric cell carcinoma with squamous cell metaplasia	20
Unspecified, undifferentiated carcinoma	95
Adenocarcinoma	21
No pathologic diagnosis available	26
Total	567

examination (table I). Some of the earliest diagnoses in this series were, in fact, obtained from incidental findings at such operations. In fact, this seems to be only possibility of getting an early diagnosis of a paranasal carcinoma.

Treatment

From the therapeutic point of view the first step in each individual case is to determine whether or not the tumor is operable. For this purpose it is important to have an opportunity to consult an otologist with extensive experience in this special field of tumor surgery.

Radiotherapy

Irradiation. In the early part of the series, radiotherapy consisted partly of conventional roentgen treatment, and partly of implantation of radium according to the technique described by BERVEN.

Roentgen treatment was usually given by four rectangular facial fields, two medial and two lateral, directing the beam towards the center of the tumor, treating 5 times weekly.

A prescribed skin exposure of about 3,000 R to each of the four fields for a period of 30 to 35 days was regarded as an adequate 'full-dose' roentgen therapy. The actual skin exposure, particularly in the anterior fields, was of course considerably higher, because of additional exposures from opposite fields.

Implantation. The other type of radiologic treatment used in 1940 to 1955 consisted of local application of radium tubes into the operative cavity in connection with electrocoagulation. As a rule four radium tubes were used, each containing 50 mg of radium. The exposure time varied from 3 to 5 hours, depending on the size of the preoperative radiation exposure. The radium tubes were usually inserted into that part of the cavity where the surgeon had felt most uncertain of the radical nature of the operation. In most cases this was the upper posterior part of the cavity. However, we have not used such local application since the end of the 1950s.

Cobalt. During the past 5 to 6 years the cobalt technique, using a total maximum exposure of 4,000 to 5,000 R in 6 weeks to two fields on the same side, has gradually been introduced.

Surgery

During the last 10 years, we have changed the surgical procedure. We use electrocoagulation very seldom and perform the operation very often by an external incision. The operative cavity is covered with skin grafts in most of our cases. In cases with tumor growing through the dura mater we resect the dura mater, and cover the defect with skin or fascia grafts.

Results of Treatment

From the therapeutic point of view, the patients can be considered as two groups: those who received radiotherapy alone, and those who received a combination of surgical treatment and radiotherapy. The absolute 5-year cure rate during the period 1940 to 1959 was 25% (148 of 591 patients).

Radiotherapy Alone
In the group that received radiotherapy alone, the 5-year cure rate was 19% (61 of 318 patients). This result may seem poor, but it should be realized that the series was limited to inoperable advanced cases in which the treatment from the beginning was considered to be merely palliative (fig. 2).

Combined Radiotherapy and Surgery
In the series of combined radiologic and surgical treatment, a 5-year cure rate of 45% was obtained.

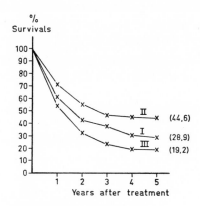

I Total series
II Combined treatment
III Radiological treatment alone

Fig. 2

The combined radiologic and operative treatment, which is dominant in this Department, is of course difficult to judge. We are very particular in calling it combination treatment and not emphasizing that it rather is a preoperative treatment. Every case is discussed in detail between the radiologist and the otologist. By the technique used at the Radiumhemmet, a very marked regression of the tumor can usually be seen during and even after the irradiation; at the following operation viable tumor is only found in about 50% of the cases in spite of the comprehensive biopsies.

Sequent Conditions

Those conditions have in part already been mentioned. Mucous membrane reactions appear during the radiation therapy and the first time afterwards, developing generally marked epithelité membranes on the mucous membranes in the nasal cavities, nasopharynx and the upper part of the mouth cavity. During this period good hygiene with regular rinses and flushings of the mouth cavity and the nasal cavities are important and will reduce the troubles for the patient. An increase in the secretions can often be noticed from the facial cavity of the affected side which regularly has been rinsed through the Caldwell-Luc opening. Later on, a mucous membrane atrophy commonly occurs and troubles the patient by the feeling of dryness and a disposition to produce dry nasty-smelling crusts in the nasal cavities and on the walls of the operative cavities. Those difficulties can be reduced through daily flushings. The skin reaction usually is confined to a vigorous dry epidermitis and perhaps a moist reaction in portions of the field.

Before concluding, we once again would like to call attention to the value of close cooperation between the otologist and the radiotherapist to obtain a good therapeutic result at cancer of the paranasal sinuses and the nasal cavities. As these tumors are relatively rare, it is advisable to concentrate the treatment to medical centers where experience then can be accumulated.

It should be borne in mind that the present series consists of unselected cases, many of them advanced, and that in all the patients who were alive at the end of the observation period the types of lesion were histologically verified.

In concluding, I would like to emphasize that our experience of the preoperative radiotherapy in cases of cancer of the paranasal sinuses and the nasal cavities is most satisfactory.

Summary

From 1940 to 1964 inclusive, 648 patients with carcinoma arising from the paranasal sinuses or the nasal cavities have been treated at the Department of Otolaryngology, Karolinska Sjukhuset, Stockholm. The treatment most frequently used was combined radiologic and surgical treatment. In the group that received such combined treatment a 5-year cure rate of 45% was obtained.

References

1. HAMBERGER, C.-A.; MÅRTENSSON, G., and SJÖGREN, H. Å.: Treatment of malignant tumors of the paranasal sinuses; in Cancer of the Head and Neck. Int. Workshop on Cancer of the Head and Neck, New York City, 1965, pp. 224–229 (Butterworths, Washington 1967).
2. LARSSON, L.-G. and MÅRTENSSON, G.: Carcinoma of the paranasal sinuses and the nasal cavities. Acta radiol. 42: 149–172 (1954).
3. LARSSON, L.-G. and MÅRTENSSON, G.: Näskaviteter och bihålor; in FEIGENBERG, POPPE and ROMANUS Strålterapi; En nordisk lärobok, pp. 216–219 (Almqvist & Wiksell, Stockholm/Göteborg/Uppsala 1963).
4. RINGERTZ, N.: Pathology of malignant tumors arising in the nasal and paranasal cavities and maxilla; med. Diss. Acta oto-laryng., Stockh., Suppl. 27 (1938).
5. ÖHNGREN, G.: Malignant tumours of the maxillo-ethmoidal region; med. Diss. Acta oto-laryng., Stockh., Suppl. 18 (1933).

Authors' address: Prof. C.-A. HAMBERGER, Department of Otolaryngology, Karolinska Sjukhuset and Prof. G. MÅRTENSSON, Department of Oral and Jaw Diseases, Karolinska Sjukhuset, S-104 01 Stockholm 60 (Sweden).

Discussion

Moderator:
ALLEN M. DEKELBOUM, M. D., Assistant Clinical Professor of Otolaryngology, University of California Medical Center, *San Francisco, Calif.*

Discussant:
RICHARD H. JESSE, Jr., M. D., Chief of Head and Neck Service, M. D. Anderson Hospital and Tumor Institute; Associate Professor of Surgery, The University of Texas, *Houston, Texas.*

JESSE: Dr. VAETH asked me to be the Devil's Advocate today. As he put it, my mission is to raise questions and to stimulate discussion.

The results presented only serve to prove that the speakers have an excellent ability to select cases which will lead to good results in their hands. Head and neck cancer patients are a curious breed of animal, with bad habits like smoking and drinking, and they rarely break these habits. Many are old and indigent, and many have other maladies, as well as cancer. We often think that we know what's best for the patient's cancer, but are often thwarted by other factors, such as his smoking and drinking, age, other diseases, socio-economic background, wants, etc. Most of us, therefore, examine the patient and his cancer, and then we select a plan of treatment aimed at getting rid of the cancer while helping the patient to stay happy and intact as possible.

The interesting thing in Dr. BILLER's paper is that they found in supraglottic and transglottic lesions, preoperative irradiation of the dose employed didn't help any, and I'd agree with this. I would ask him, how do they select their patients? They had, as I remember, 120 preops and 172 that didn't have any irradiation. Since he states that supraglottic and transglottic cancers are not helped by his dose of irradiation, does he now, today, use it? He's reported a dose of 1,500 to 3,000 rads, and that's quite a difference; I don't know whether it was an average or whether most of it was somewhere in the middle. None of these patients are staged in his report, and the interesting thing, I thought, were his figures for the pyriform sinus and base of tongue, which showed a 48% three-year survival. His local recurrence rate was 18% and his neck recurrence rate was 23%. Our own figures in 157 patients showed the same local recurrence rate and the same neck recurrence rate, but our 3-year survival rate is only 30%, instead of 48%. I think the reason is that we probably see more late disease, as we have a 19% distant metastases rate, which is a good deal higher than that reported here today.

In Dr. SILVERSTONE's and Dr. GOLDMAN's papers, I'm a little confused as to whether they included the entire population of their institutions in their series. If so, 53 patients in the number of years that they said, is not a great number of patients for an active service. Are these patients force-fed during their radiation therapy? Because all of their patients healed, and all of my patients don't heal. I want to know how they accomplished this. Are they kept in the hospital? What is the percentage of postoperative fistulas? I know they all healed eventually, but how many of them broke down? Was there any fatality in the series at all? Apparently not, but I wasn't sure.

The interesting thing here is that they have a 10% local failure rate. I have a 14% local failure rate in our combined series of 49 patients, and a 15% local recurrence rate in 103 surgically-treated patients. This is a 24% local recurrence rate in 115 patients treated by irradiation, but I hasten to add that half of these can be salvaged by surgery later on. The interesting thing is that the rate of absolute survival in this paper was, as I remember, 79%, and in our series it's 64%. Now, this can mean only one thing to me: we're still comparing the same patients, because 15% of our patients will be dead of distant metastases within that two-year period, so I couldn't possibly get anything but somewhere below 85%, just on this basis alone. There must be a difference of groups.

Dr. HENDRICKSON's paper was an interesting study, comparing 2,000 rads and 5,000 rads preoperatively, and the results were the same, therefore concluding that high and low dose irradiation were equal. Of 59 patients, 51 were supraglottic larynx lesions. Both Dr. BILLER and I agree that this is a poor choice because it doesn't make any difference whether you give them any irradiation or not at any level. There were 36 N_0's and 14 N_1's, and only 9 N_2's in the study, with a 76% two-year survival in the N_0 group. Now I can show you a 75% cure rate in the irradiation-alone group, without any surgery in the supraglottic larynx. So I would really question whether preoperative irradiation in the pure supraglottic group is worthwhile at all. I don't question, however, that it is worthwhile in base of tongue, pyriform sinus, pharyngeal wall, and oropharynx, but I think in the supraglottic lesion, one must be careful to compare this with a good irradiation-alone or surgery-alone series, or maybe both.

Dr. HAMBERGER's paper is a tremendous series. His figures are exactly the same as mine, almost to within 2% for both his raw survival rate, and his so-called curable cases, somewhere in the neighborhood of 45%. He does, however, have 74 cylindromas in the group, which I would submit have a pretty good 5-year survival rate.

I hope that my discussion, rather than being vitriolic, which it is not intended to be, does raise some questions, and I hope that both the speakers and the audience will participate in a discussion at this time.

GALANTE: The only thing I can say about Dr. JESSE's remarks is this: I remember being in a symposium with him several years ago, and he was very enthusiastic and looking forward to randomized series. It appears to me that he has lost his enthusiasm for this type of study. I don't know whether this type of study can be carefully carried out, with large numbers of cases. I also don't think that we will resolve the problem of comparable patients, as all of our work is selection. There is no question about it; we select cases. I think that the problem is one of deciding if there is a class of lesions where preoperative radiation therapy is going to be effective? And if so, how should this preoperative radiation therapy be given, to what extent, in what doses, and in what time? It would be very difficult to obtain similar patients for all groups, Dr. JESSE. I just don't know how that could be done.

BILLER: I'd like to thank Dr. JESSE for his comments. There's no doubt that in a retrospective study there's always room for great criticism. But I think that in reviewing a retrospective study you can get some valid information which will enable you to establish a better prospective study. I think that is so in this one.

As far as the patients that died of intercurrent disease, which were equally divided between the preoperative and the non-preoperative groups, 18 out of the patients have autopsies without evidence of recurrent tumor. This created a dilemma, so we elected to delete them, whether this is acceptable or not.

The preoperative irradiation study at Washington University was started about 1961 or 1962, and initially there was a problem as to how much to give, 1,500 rads or 3,000 rads. About 80% of these patients presented today received 3,000 rads, and the rest 1,500 rads with a few that had 2,000 rads. The selection of patients likewise was dictated by the fact that since 1962 about 95% of the patients with these lesions were preoperatively irradiated.

We are now in the process, with Dr. PEREZ and Dr. POWERS, of starting a prospective study. The prospective study is not going to include supraglottic lesions because we feel there is enough evidence that preoperative irradiation does not add anything there. In our study 1,500 rads did not change the neck recurrence rate, and so we feel that after looking at Dr. GOLDMAN's results, it could be that if we were to give 5,000 rads to the neck with little or no dose to the primary we could still increase the survival rate for supraglottic lesions.

The only reason that we did not take the epiglottic lesions and divide them into T_1 and T_2 was that by so doing we would have broken down the population so small that one could not draw anything from it.

We feel that pyriform sinus lesions can be cured, judging from our results and those of SOM, GOLDMAN and CHAMBERS, and that there is enough evidence even retrospectively to indicate that preoperative irradiation is beneficial. When one starts to establish a protocol at this time I think it's necessary to look back in the literature and see what other people are doing, because I personally would be very hesitant to take a pyriform sinus lesion and on the basis of a protocol treat with X-ray alone. I certainly would be just as hesitant to treat a pyriform sinus lesion with surgery alone. I think there's enough evidence which supports that preoperative irradiation is beneficial in decreasing local recurrence and thereby enhancing survival to indicate that it should be given. Now, the major question is the dose, and I think that this is what should be randomized.

As far as the complications, I just want to make one point. In all the cases that I've seen, the incidence of complications is no higher with high doses, but the complications with the higher doses are more disastrous, once they occur.

GOLDMAN: I would like to congratulate the organizing committee for arranging this symposium. I believe it's the first of its kind where the whole subject of combined therapy is discussed in this fashion. I wouldn't want to leave unless we reach some conclusions which are reasonable and can lead us in a direction which will provide the best care for patients with these terrible diseases.

I'm a little concerned about statements that are being made. In the first place, I have had tremendous exposure to the practice of radiotherapy, and I have great faith in radiotherapy. I believe that radiotherapy is one of the best conservative measures of treating cancer of the larynx. With Dr. SILVERSTONE, we have treated hundreds of T_1 and T_2 cancers of the larynx by radiotherapy, and I dare say that our statistics are as good as any by surgery. So we are very much sympathetic towards radiotherapy. And by the way, a T_2N_0 lesion of the epiglottis we would treat with radiotherapy. We wouldn't include that in our series. And as I'm on the subject, the cases in this series are patients supervised entirely by me and they are consecutive cases.

T_1N_0, T_2N_0 cases are treated entirely by radiotherapy. But once you get beyond that stage, it becomes a surgical problem. I don't see why this patient can't get the benefit of the best there is, and the best there is is the combination. We must be ready to accept combined therapy as an evolutionary step in the treatment of cancer of the upper respiratory tract. Yes, it may require us as surgeons to be more careful, to be more fastidious, to employ certain particular techniques, etc. Perhaps in some instances we did get increased complications and that patient's stay in the hospital was longer, but in the end, every patient survived. Every patient left the hospital in good shape.

We have 53 patients, having undergone 90 procedures. There were 41 complications, including 10 wound infections. If there was any stitch abcess at the edge of the wound, or a little exudate, that's included as an infection. Six patients had pharyngeal strictures, which is overemphasized as it is merely the tightness into the esophagus and all these patients were well handled by dilatation. This hemorrhage that we spoke of was a non-carotid hemorrhage, a vessel which was easily controlled. We had 4 carotid exposures, no blow-outs, we had 8 flaps, 4 for the carotids and 4 for fistulas. There were 19 fistulas. All these patients healed. Was there an increase in complications? I will grant the possibility that there was an increase. A serious increase? I question this. I've been practicing a long time. I remember these patients before the days of antibiotics and radiotherapy, and as many of you know, we had our share of fistulas in T_4 lesions, and laryngeal-pharyngeal lesions. So I don't think that is a critical point. What is a critical point is that in the Stage IV lesions you triple your survival rate. How can anybody deny this? By great skill of surgery? No. Every one of these cases was operated by a resident with my assistance. And the statisticians tell us that if you have 50 cases and if you more than double your survival rate, then this increase is statistically valid. And this is in reference to the need of creating controls to make this work valid. If you go through the literature for the last 20 years or more, there are plenty of cases for comparison: the T, N, M system is not perfect, but it's fairly good, and it gives you a means of some comparison. There are thousands of cases now that have been treated by surgery alone, by irradiation alone, etc. and these are adequate controls. How can we start a controlled study now, after what we've seen? You can sacrifice hamsters for controls, but I'm not going to sacrifice human beings for controls, when I can triple their survival rate. I think that is ethically wrong.

As I said before, for the T_1N_0 and T_2N_0 lesions, we treat with irradiation alone, but this isn't the challenge. With the combined approach with Stage II cases – that's T_3N_0 and T_4N_0 lesions – we have 100% control rate in three years (10 out of 10). Now that must germinate ideas in your minds. This is where we should be heading. So the thought I would like to leave with you is that we've come to this meeting for a purpose, and we have such a highly talented group here, an interested group, that I would hope that we could arrive at constructive conclusions. And I think one of the constructive conclusions is that high dosage irradiation is not any more dangerous than low dosage irradiation, and it produces far better results.

JESSE: Here's the figure I can't figure out right here: when I have 15% distant metastases, I just don't know how you can get that figure. That would put that figure for me down to 85%, meaning nobody can die of anything else except distant metastases.

GOLDMAN: There were three cases of metastases. I think one case of metastasis existed prior to surgery, which we didn't pick up.

JESSE: How many pyriform sinuses are in your study?

GOLDMAN: The Stage IV cases are all advanced laryngo-pharyngeal cases. They're practically all pyriform sinuses.

JESSE: What percentage of them had positive nodes?

GOLDMAN: It's a good question. I can't give you the precise answer, but it was quite high, perhaps 65–80%.

JESSE: I'm not arguing; I think you're right as far as your 5,000 rads preop irradiation is concerned, but I don't want to be misunderstood. I am worried about the figures. I just don't know how they can be quite that good.

GOLDMAN: Why not?

JESSE: Because I don't think anybody in the country could get that survival.

GOLDMAN: I didn't get the figure, we just added it up. And Dr. JESSE, I was as surprised as you are.

JESSE: I congratulate you.

GOLDMAN: Don't congratulate me, congratulate combined therapy, 5,500 rads, and good surgery. That's all there is to it. We came up with an idea, we followed it through honestly and logically to the letter, and that is it. There are absolutely correct statistics.

JESSE: I'm not arguing about that; the thing I'm arguing about is, are these cases absolutely Stage III and IV?

GOLDMAN: All the evidence, as of today, shows that low dosage irradiation has been a failure, particularly in preventing local recurrence. Dr. STRONG, from Memorial Hospital, admitted to me that they're through with low dosage, because he had 22% recurrence rate in the neck. And we've had none. So let us, as a group of doctors, come to a conclusion and follow through on this.

FLETCHER: We must invite Dr. GOLDMAN to come to the M. D. ANDERSON Hospital, and he will see that anywhere from 10–20% of our patients are absolutely inoperable, regardless of preoperative irradiation, 1,500–10,000 rads. We have right there a palliative group. Now, where is a palliative group in Dr. GOLDMAN's series? Secondly, we have, as previously mentioned, approximately a 20% incidence of distant metastases. Thirdly, most of our patients are 65 years or older. 15 or 20% die from intercurrent disease. The very best we could hope to achieve would be a 60% cure rate. We frequently review our tonsil material, and we have approximately 50% alive at five years. Of the 50% dead, only 20% died with disease above the clavicle. It is absolutely remarkable that you have only 3 patients with distant metastases, and finally 90% local control. The Biblical days have come back.

DEKELBOUM: I might interject one thought: What role, I wonder, does preoperative radiation therapy have in reducing distant metastases? Perhaps this might account for the differential that one sees in the 15% that Dr. JESSE talks about. Before we get more involved with this heated discussion we should give Dr. HENDRICKSON an opportunity to speak.

HENDRICKSON: There are several things that are important to point out. First: Yes, Dr. JESSE, we would like very much to treat the T_3N_0 patients with radiotherapy alone. However, if our surgeons feel that they are sufficiently advanced lesions, then they would like to operate on them. This is one of the areas in which there are legitimate differences of opinion, and I think they will always exist. We should all recognize that the American Joint Committee on Staging & End Results Reporting have defined methods of staging and methods of end results reporting, and I don't think anybody here today used the methods suggested by the committee. I would submit that the suggested methods contain the appropriate ways of handling patients dying of intercurrent disease. They also contain appropriate ways of handling patients who are lost to follow-up. If we would all be consistent and follow what we had at one time worked out, we might be better able to compare the things that we are discussing so heatedly today. Lastly, Dr. FLETCHER came to the crux of the matter when he commented that many patients do die of distant metastases, and possibly when we're talking about combined forms of treatment our end points should not be life or death. Again, as Dr. ROTKIN this morning suggested, there are many variables that influence clinical trials and possibly we should be assessing the effects of the treatment on the part of the body that was treated. Some patients die of distant disease, but it doesn't negate the effects of the treatment on the part of the body that was treated. I would hope that the prospective study that our colleagues in Chicago have agreed to will ultimately answer some of the questions that were raised here. There are now a number of patients in that study which does have a surgery-only control. This has been very difficult because Dr. GOLDMAN, for instance, was already convinced that preoperative radiotherapy was a benefit and he'll not permit his patients to undergo surgery alone. We have excluded the hypopharynx and pyriform fossa lesions from the study because we also feel that these all should get preoperative radiotherapy. I think it's unfair to take the lesion that is overwhelmingly laryngeal, but because it creeps over the aryepiglottic fold and down the one side of the pyriform fossa, and to then say that this is a pyriform fossa lesion. We should still stage disease by where the tumor seems to arise.

Front. Radiation Ther. Onc., vol. 5, pp. 147–154
(Karger, Basel/München/Paris/New York 1970)

Combined Radiation and Surgical Treatment of Carcinoma of the Thoracic Esophagus

R. L. SCOTTE DOGGETT, III[1], JAMES M. GUERNSEY[2]
and MALCOLM A. BAGSHAW[3]

The results of surgical and radiation therapy alone in the treatment of patients with thoracic esophageal cancer at Stanford Medical Center have been poor. Only five of 65 patients (8%) survived without evidence of disease for over two years following 5500 rads or more to the tumor and what appeared radiographically to be adequate margins. An analysis of autopsies performed on 45 of these patients showed that 58% died with tumor confined to the esophagus and/or the regional nodes in the epigastrium. This high incidence of local failure of radiation treatment and the poor surgical experience (3) resulted in the Division of Radiation Therapy and Department of Surgery undertaking this clinical investigation.

Materials and Methods

Forty-two patients were included in the investigation, 28 males and 14 females. Forty-one patients had squamous cancers; one patient had an adenocarcinoma which was clearly demonstrated to arise from the lower third of the esophagus at the time of abdominal exploration. Patients were excluded only if hemato-

[1] Assistant Professor, Department of Radiology, Division of Radiation Therapy, Stanford University School of Medicine; since September, 1969, Radiation Therapy Center, 1215 Twenty-eighth Street, Sacramento, CA 95816.

[2] Assistant Professor, Department of Surgery, Stanford University School of Medicine; currently with U.S. Army Medical Corps.

[3] Professor, Department of Radiology, Division of Radiation Therapy, Stanford University School of Medicine.

genous metastases were detected or if it was determined by the surgical consultant that there were medical contraindications to esophagectomy. Five patients were excluded for medical reasons. Old age alone was not a contraindication to combined therapy; four patients were 70 years of age or older (average age 61 years).

All patients underwent upper abdominal exploration and had gastrostomies. At the time of exploration, suspicious perigastric and/or celiac nodes were biopsied; random node biopsies were carried out if enlarged nodes were not present. Care was taken to position the gastrostomy out of the epigastric field of radiation therapy. Patients with upper and middle third lesions underwent bronchoscopy. Scalene node biopsies were done only when there was clinical suspicion of involvement.

All patients were treated on the 6-MeV linear accelerator. Midplane doses of 3500–4400 rads were delivered to the entire esophagus in all patients. Patients with mid- and lower-third tumors received the same dose to the epigastrium, a field including the celiac axis and proximal third of the stomach. The initial 3500–4400 rads were delivered through single, matched, antero-posterior fields which included the medial supraclavicular fossae in all patients. Supplemental doses of 1500–2200 rads were directed to the primary tumor with 4 cm margins using rotational or oblique field techniques to avoid the spinal cord. The total tumor dose was 5000 rads in 11 and 6600 rads in 31 patients. If subdiaphragmatic nodes were involved, a total dose of 6000 rads was delivered to the mid-plane of the epigastrium. Patients were treated four times a week, 250–275 rads to the mid-plane per treatment. No correction for lung transmission was made.

Patients were reevaluated for metastatic disease four – five weeks following completion of radiation therapy. Patients under-went upper abdominal exploration followed by total esophagec-tomy if hematogenous metastases were not detected and the epigastrium and liver were found to be free of tumor. Stomach or colon interposition was carried out at the same stage as esopha-gectomy. Esophageal replacement with stomach was used in 14 of 22 patients; the anastomosis was developed above the media-stinum when possible.

Results

Twenty-two of 42 patients completed the planned radiation therapy, esophagectomy and interposition (table I). In two patients, radiation therapy was not completed because of a massive pulmonary infarction and development of a broncho-esophageal fistula. Eleven patients were not submitted to surgery. Fistula formation between the esophagus and major airways occurred in three patients; two patients had massive hemorrhages as a result of erosion of the aorta by tumor. Four patients had distant metastases when reevaluated following radiation therapy. One patient was not operated because of palpable epigastric nodes. Radiation pneumonitis prevented surgery in one patient. Five patients were operated but did not undergo esophagectomy. Two of these had lung metastases detected at surgery; one had persistent epigastric node involvement; two patients had tracheo-esophageal fistulae which proved to be non-resectable. Two patients underwent partial resection in an effort to palliate advanced residual tumor; interposition was not attempted in these patients. All patients failing to complete combined radiation-surgical treatment had either local and/or metastatic tumor at postmortem.

Celiac and/or perigastric node biopsies were carried out in 37 of 42 patients. Included were six of seven patients with upper third primary tumors, 20 of 23 with mid third and 11 of 12 with lower third segment tumors. The biopsies were positive in none of the upper, nine (45%) of the mid, and six (55%) of the lower third lesions. Supraclavicular node involvement was present in three patients, including one with an upper third segment tumor and two with mid third tumors (both patients had epigastric nodes

Table I. Preoperative radiation and surgical treatment of cancer of the thoracic esophagus

	No.	%
Patients starting treatment	42	100
Radiation Rx completed	40	95
Esophagectomy attempted	29	69
Esophagectomy accomplished	24	57
Esophagectomy and interposition	22	52
Alive without disease (60 & 32 mos)	2	5

involved as well). Four of 16 patients with epigastric node involvement had microscopic spread of tumor which was not anticipated by the surgeon who had carried out a random node biopsy.

Two of 22 patients who completed combination therapy are surviving without evidence of tumor for over two years (table II). Fatal complications within 30 days occurred in eight of 24 patients (33%) undergoing esophagectomy. Three patients had gastro-esophago-tracheal fistulae. A single patient died of each of the following complications: Interposed colon necrosis, broncho-pleural fistula, massive pleural bleeding, pneumothorax, and empyema. No tumor was found at autopsy in four of the eight patients suffering fatal surgical complications.

Radiation therapy complications proved fatal in five of 40 patients (12.5%). Though elements of both pericardial and myo-cardial fibrosis were present in four patients, pericardial fibrosis was thought to be the primary cause of death in two patients (seven and 25 months following institution of treatment), while complications of myocardial fibrosis resulted in the death of two patients (25 and 69 months after treatment). One patient died of acute radiation pneumonitis three months following institution of radiation treatment.

Table II. Results of preoperative radiotherapy, total esophagectomy and interposition 22 patients

Alive without tumor	2	(60, 32 mos)
Fatal complications	12	
Surgical		8
Radiation		4[1]
Dead of disease	8	

[1]Ned at 7, 25, 25 & 69 mos

Discussion

This limited investigation emphasizes the value of surgical staging in planning therapy of patients with cancer of the thoracic esophagus. Upper abdominal exploration with biopsy of lymph nodes and liver along with gastrostomy was carried out without major complication. There is a direct relationship between the extent of disease and survival as shown in table III. There were no survivors in patients with proven involvement of the bronchus, trachea, or recurrent laryngeal nerve (T4), or in patients with proven involvement of extrathoracic nodes, either supraclavicular or subdiaphragmatic (N3). In four patients who died of distant metastases, involvement of epigastric nodes could not be detected at the time of esophagectomy or at autopsy, though tumor had been proven to be present before radiation therapy. Upper abdominal exploration is advised in patients with carcinomas of the mid and lower segments of the esophagus. Combined radiation and surgical therapy is reserved for patients with tumors in Stage I

Table III. Results of planned combined radiation and surgical treatment two years survival vs extent of disease

	N_0 No nodes	N_1 Adjacent thoracic	N_2 Distant thoracic	N_3 Extrathoracic
T_1 5 cm or less	2/7[1] 3/9 Stage I	1/2		0/1
T_2 5–10 cm	1/9 1/10 Stage II	0/1	1/4	0/9
T_3 10 cm +	0/1 1/5 Stage III			0/1
T_4 Bronch., Trach., Laryn. N.	0/2 0/18 Stage IV			0/5

[1] NED 2 years + / Total patients

through III. Although the experience is limited, involvement of mediastinal lymph nodes other than those adjacent to the esophagus (N2) is not a contraindication to combined treatment.

Twenty-two of 40 patients (55%) completing radiation therapy underwent curative esophagectomy and reconstruction. This suggests a favorable effect of radiation, as few institutions report resectability rates over 40% when tumors at all levels are considered. Furthermore, the likelihood of survival appears related to the effects of radiation on the resected primary tumor. Four surgical specimens were tumor free, while ten had microscopic and eight had gross residual tumor. Ten of the 14 patients with no tumor or microscopic tumor are alive, or dead of complications without cancer, including five patients surviving over two years. All eight patients with gross residual tumor in the resected specimen died with cancer; five patients had tumor in the bed of the esophagus while seven had hematogenous spread of disease.

The surgical mortality rate varies with the level of the tumor; however, various authors report overall operative mortality rates averaging 20%. The higher rate in this series (33%) may relate to the preoperative radiation therapy. Paramediastinal radiation pneumonitis and chronic pleural effusions exaggerate the postoperative ventilatory problems imposed by one-stage esophagectomy and reconstruction in debilitated patients, many of whom had significant emphysema. This was most evident in three patients who had pneumothorax postoperatively. Prolonged use of chest tubes was necessary to bring about lung re-expansion in two patients; pneumothorax was eventually fatal in the third. Breakdown of the esophago-gastric anastomosis was fatal in three patients. The detrimental effects of radiation on healing of anastomoses are well recognized and probably played a role in this complication. Two major changes in treatment protocol may decrease the incidence of this complication. The dose of radiation to the epigastrium and cervical esophagus is significantly reduced and esophagectomy and interposition is being carried out in two stages. A minimum of three months elapses between esophagectomy and reconstruction. This results in a decrease in the operating time, allows for improvement in the general nutritional and pulmonary status, and provides further time to detect metastatic disease and thus avoid unnecessary surgery. Surgical considerations have been discussed more completely by one of us (J. M. G.) elsewhere (2).

Radiation morbidity and mortality were excessive. Fatal radiation pneumonitis occurred in a patient who had emphysema and an exaggerated thoracic kyphosis which made it difficult to avoid treating the spinal cord without using posterior oblique fields which traversed considerable lung tissue. Pericardial and myocardial injury by radiation is related directly to the volume of heart radiated and to the dose delivered (4). The incidence of cardiac complications of radiation therapy may not be appreciated as is suggested in this experience. Two patients, ages 75 and 54 years, died 25 and 69 months following institution of combined therapy. Postmortem examinations were carried out at other institutions without the knowledge that high dose radiation therapy had been given. Pathological diagnoses of congestive heart failure secondary to arteriosclerotic heart disease were made. Review of the pathological material showed diffuse interstitial fibrosis associated with radiation injury (1). Cardiac complications are of particular significance, having occurred in four patients who had no tumor at postmortem examination nine, 25, 25 and 69 months following institution of radiation treatment.

Changes have been made to decrease both surgical and radiation complications. The dose to the entire esophagus has been decreased to 3500 rads over a four-week interval. An additional increment of 1500 rads is directed to the tumor with radiographically normal appearing esophagus 4 cm above and below in a two-week treatment time. Four of 16 patients had random epigastric node biopsies which were positive, suggesting a higher incidence of involvement than we have shown. For this reason, the epigastrium is treated to a mid-plane dose of 3500 rads in four weeks in patients with tumors arising from the mid and lower segments.

Summary

Forty-two patients with carcinoma of the thoracic esophagus were included in a program of upper abdominal exploration, gastrostomy, preoperative radiation therapy and one-stage esophagectomy and interposition. Treatment was completed in 22 patients, two of whom are alive without evidence of disease. In analyzing treatment failures, it was concluded that no patient benefited from combined therapeutic approach when the primary tumor was proven to involve adjacent mediastinal structures or had metastasized to epigastric nodes. Lower doses of radiation and two-stage eso-phagectomy-reconstruction procedures are advised to reduce the incidence of major complications.

References

1. FAJARDO, L. F.; STEWART, J. R., and COHN, K. E.: Morphology of radiation-induced heart disease. Arch. Path. *86* : 513–519 (1968).
2. GUERNSEY, J. M.; DOGGETT, R. L. S.; MASON, G. R.; KOHATSU, S., and OBERHELMAN, H. A.: Combined treatment of cancer of the esophagus. Amer. J. Surg. *117:* 157–161 (1969).
3. KAY, S.: A ten-year appraisal of the treatment of squamous cell carcinoma of the esophagus. Surg. Gynec. Obstet. *117:* 167 (1963).
4. STEWART, J. R.; COHN, K. E.; FAJARDO, L. J.; HANCOCK, E. W., and KAPLAN, H. S.: Radiation-induced heart disease. Radiology *89 :* 302–310 (1967).

Authors' addresses: R. L. SCOTTE DOGGETT, III, MD, Radiation Therapy Center, 1215 Twenty-eighth Street, *Sacramento, CA 95816*; JAMES M. GUERNSEY, MD, Department of Surgery and MALCOLM A. BAGSHAW, MD, Department of Radiology, Division of Radiation Therapy, Stanford University School of Medicine, *Palo Alto, Cal.* (USA).

Front. Radiation Ther. Onc., vol. 5, pp. 155–162
(Karger, Basel/München/Paris/New York 1970)

High Dose Preoperative Radiation Therapy in Carcinoma of the Rectosigmoid Colon

C. V. ALLEN

Department of Radiation Therapy, University of Oregon Medical School, Portland, Ore.

Carcinoma of the colon is second only to lung in mortality from malignancy. There has been no improvement in survival since 1940 with 21% to 34% 5-year survival in all cases, and 38% to 60% with 'curative operable' cases. Seventy percent of colon malignancies are in the lower 25 cm.

Although LEAMING [4] reported better results in Dukes's Class C lesions with low dose preoperative radiation, ROSWIT [7] was not able to confirm this in a large well controlled series. High dose local irradiation with radium preoperatively has been reported by RUFF [8]. More recently TEPPER [9] and his group described their early experience with nineteen patients given external irradiation in the order of 4,500 R in 4½ weeks.

In May 1960 a decision was made at the University of Oregon Medical School to give higher dose preoperative irradiation to adenocarcinoma of the rectosigmoid than had been previously reported. The purpose of this study was to determine patient tolerance to such irradiation, evaluate changes in surgical complications, test the possibility of converting unresectable to resectable lesions, and assess changes in survival and survival patterns. This was considered a phase I feasibility study and there was no randomization of cases. However, cases at the Veterans Administration Hospital managed by the same surgical and radiotherapy staff were to be treated with surgery only, and later used as a comparison group.

The protocol agreed upon by the Departments of Surgery and Radiation Therapy specified abdominal exploration for assessment of metastases and unresectability, plus establishment of a colostomy to divert the fecal stream from an area that might not tolerate both high dose irradiation and the usual passage of stool. This was to be followed by 5,000 R delivered to the primary tumor. Definitive surgery, usually abdominal perineal resection, was to follow four or five weeks later. After a year of experience with the study, colostomy was no longer considered necessary as a routine, and was done only in cases of obstruction. Patients were excluded who had recognized metastases, history of previous irradiation, poor general condition, colostomy stoma within the field, bowel obstruction (colostomy mandatory) or infection such as diverticulitis, cystitis, etc. Unresectability due to fixation was not a cause for rejection.

All patients were treated with the 2MEV Van de Graaff generator at 100 cm or telecobalt at 80 cm. Most patients were treated through opposing anterior and posterior fields, others with low lying lesions were treated with various combinations of anterior, posterior and perineal fields utilizing wedge filters. Localizing films were obtained in all except perineal fields. The rate of treatment was 900 R per week. Because lymphatic metastases often fail to progress in an orderly fashion [1] resulting in frequent skip areas and unpredictable location of involved nodes, no attempt was made to include lymphatic drainage areas in the treatment field. Fields encompassing all potentially involved intra-abdominal lymphatics would be larger than we believed prudent to treat and would include the duodenum. Relatively small fields, usually 10×10 cm were designed to include the primary tumor only and spare the normal tissue as much as possible.

Table I. Rectosigmoid Ca

Study cases	73
Irradiation and surgery	52
Irradiation only	21

Material

Seventy-three patients have been entered into the study. Eighteen of these were unresectable prior to irradiation because of fixation of tumor. Fifty-two were irradiated and resected, the remaining 21 received irradiation only and were not resected because of the appearence of metastases, patient refusal, or failure to convert an unresectable lesion to resectable (table I).

Complications

Tolerance to treatment was good. The few cases of diarrhea were controlled with Paregoric and diet. There were no significant depressions of blood count, and the only notable surface reaction occurred when colostomy stoma or mucous fistula was in the treatment field. Ulceration occurred at about 3,500 R. This was corrected by changing from anterior and posterior fields, to posterior and perineal. In one patient the mucous fistula was replaced prior to irradiation.

Spontaneous rupture of the colon occurred post irradiation in two of the 73 patients.

Technical problems at surgery were not increased by pre-operative irradiation except in one case where the dose was carried well above the 5,000 R prescribed. Postoperative complications are listed in table II.

Results

Unresectable lesions. As listed in table III 18 patients were deemed unresectable prior to irradiation, and nine of these became resectable. Of these nine, six died with carcinoma, one is alive

Table II. Postoperative complications rectosigmoid carcinoma

	Preop. irradiation	Surgery only[1]
Abscesses	6%	9%
Wound healing	13%	18%

[1] (2).

with, and two alive without carcinoma. Of those remaining unresectable three are dead with carcinoma, five alive with carcinoma up to 60 months, and one alive without carcinoma (table III).

Table III. Unresectable rectosigmoid carcinoma

18 cases irradiated:
9 became resectable
    6 – dead with ca
    1 – alive with ca
    2 – no evidence of disease
9 remained unresectable
    3 – dead with ca
    5 – alive with ca up to 60 months
    1 – no evidence of disease

Sterilization of carcinoma. In the 52 surgical specimens five were free of carcinoma and five exhibited only *in situ* carcinoma. Nine of the ten patients are alive without carcinoma, and one dead of intercurrent disease (table IV).

Table IV. Tumor sterilization – rectosigmoid Ca

In situ   5
No ca   5
    9 – alive without ca
    1 – dead intercurrent disease

Survival. Comparing this study group with a previously un-irradiated series there is no difference in survival at 2 years (table V).

Table V. Two-year tumor-free survival – rectosigmoid Ca

Surgery only[1]	70/101 (70%)
Irradiation & Surgery	25/36 (69%)

[1] (2).

Local recurrences. There has been no clinical evidence of local recurrence in 52 cases.

Influence of colostomy. At the present time our data indicate that patients without pre-irradiation colostomy have a better survival rate than those with colostomy as shown on table VI. It is recognized that the series is too small for final conclusion. Duke's method of staging has been utilized realizing that his classification is based on surgical findings and therefore not strictly applicable to preoperative situations.

Table VI. Survival relative to colostomy

	Colostomy	No colostomy
Stage I	3/7 (42%)	14/16 (87%)
Stage II	3/9 (33%)	7/9 (77%)
Stage III	3/6 (50%)	4/5 (80%)
Total	9/22 (48%)	25/30 (80%)

Lymph nodes. Apparently viable neoplasm was found in the lymph nodes from eleven of the 52 surgical specimens. Three of these patients are alive without disease up to 48 months, two dead of intercurrent disease, one alive with and five dead with carcinoma.

Discussion

As anticipated, the tolerance to this dose of irradiation was good. The cause of the two spontaneous colon ruptures in 73 cases is unclear. The first occurred at five weeks post-irradiation and autopsy was denied. Cause of the death was peritonitis. The second perforation was an incidental finding at post mortem with cerebral vascular accident listed as the cause of death. The perforation was found proximal to the tumor and probably out of the treatment field. Spontaneous colon perforation does occur in patients with bowel malignancies who have not had irradiation, therefore we do not confirm or deny irradiation as a factor in these two accidents.

Our surgeons report hyperemia in an occasional case at surgery and increased fibrosis if there has been previous surgery. An anastomotic leak and abscess formation occurred in one of the five patients having anterior resection. One or both of the anastomotic ends may have been in the treatment field. When anterior resection rather than abdominal perineal resection is anticipated, careful planning to spare anastomotic ends from irradiation seems critical. The incidence of three postoperative abscesses in 52 cases is less than in a previous series with 15 abscesses occurring in 162 patients having had surgery alone. Wound healing problems were not increased and postoperative complications in this series are fewer than in the previously un-irradiated series.

Of the 18 locally fixed, unresectable lesions, nine became resectable post-irradiation. Two of the nine are apparently free of tumor at 5 and 12 months. One that remained unresectable appears to be tumor-free at 45 months. It appears that some patients with unresectable tumor can be salvaged with the combined therapy approach.

Although only one of the larger tumors was sterilized, ten of the 52 surgical specimens contained only *in situ* or no carcinoma. No evidence of metastases has occurred in these ten patients, and those with microfocal or no carcinoma in the specimen seem to have an unusually good prognosis.

It is inappropriate in this phase of the study to make conclusions regarding influence of combined therapy on survival. There is no difference at the 2-year level comparing this study with the previously unirradiated series from our Institution. The absence of local recurrence in 52 cases is believed significant. GILCHRIST [3] and MORGAN [5] have found an approximate 22% local recurrence after surgery alone, and REYNOLDS [6] lists this as the most common cause of postoperative failure.

Such recurrences are usually evident within the first 2 years after surgery [10]. If further experience substantiates a marked decrease in local recurrence, we believe this should be reflected in an improved 5-year survival that would not be apparent at the 2-year period.

Pre-irradiation colostomy was mandatory in the first period of our study. We later doubted the necessity of the procedure except with complete obstruction, and after the first year few patients were subjected to the procedure. On reviewing the data we were surprised to see better survival in patients without colostomy. This difference did not seem to be related to stage of disease. Salvage was poorer in all stages with pre-irradiation colostomy. Theoretically, if the difference is valid, trauma to the liver and manipulation of the primary tumor showering the lymphatic and blood vascular system with tumor cells may be a factor in the differential survival. Postoperative decrease in host resistance to tumor must also be considered. Cause of death in the failures was distant metastases and not local recurrence.

We have also irradiated four patients with partial obstruction without benefit of pre-irradiation colostomy. Two of these obstructions cleared with irradiation, in one there was no change, and the obstruction became complete in the fourth requiring colostomy. Only one treatment day was lost because of surgery.

Summary

Seventy-three patients have been entered in a study of preoperative radiation for carcinoma of the rectosigmoid colon. Observations after the first nine years are considered preliminary but seem to indicate that tumor doses in the order of 5,000 R in 5½ weeks are well tolerated and have not increased complications. Some unresectable lesions became resectable. No clinical evidence of local recurrence has been found in fifty-two patients having completed combined treatment, and the patients without preoperative colostomy seem to do better than those with colostomy. We hope a cooperative study will materialize for obtaining more meaningful data.

References

1. COLLER, F. A.: Cancer of the colon and rectum (Monograph) American Cancer Society, Inc. 1956.
2. FLETCHER, W. S.; KRIPPAEHNE, W. W.; HARDWICK, C. E., and DUNPHY, J. E.: Carcinoma of the colon and rectum. Results of treatment in a County Hospital population. Amer. J. Surg. *105:* 117 (1963).
3. GILCHRIST, R. K. and DAVID, V. C.: Consideration of pathological factors influencing 5-year survival in radical resection of large bowel and rectum for carcinoma. Ann. Surg. *126:* 421 (1947).
4. LEAMING, R. H.; STEARNS, M. W., and DEDDISH, M. R.: Preoperative Irradiation in Rectal Carcinoma. Radiology *77:* 257 (1961).
5. MORGAN, C. N.: Discussion on major surgery in carcinoma of the rectum with or without colostomy, excluding the anal canal and including the rectosigmoid: Restorative resection. Proc. Roy. Soc. Med. *50:* 1,050 (1957).

6. REYNOLDS, C. T.; LA COSTE, C. E.; ROGERS, P. R., Jr., and YATSHUHASHI, M.: Total salvage in adenocarcinoma of the rectum and rectosigmoid. Surg. Gynec. Obstet. *127:* 975 (1968).

7. ROSWIT, B. and HIGGINS, G.: Personal communications.

8. RUFF, C. C.; DOCKERTY, M. B.; FRICK, R. E., and WAUGH J., M.: Preoperative radiation therapy for adenocarcinoma of the rectum and rectosigmoid. Surg. Gynec. Obstet. *112:* 715 (1961).

9. TEPPER, M.; VIDONE, R. A.; HAYES, M. A.; LINDENMUTH, W. W., and KLIGERMAN, M. W.: Preoperative irradiation in rectal cancer: initial comparison of clinical tolerance, surgical and pathologic findings. Amer. J. Roentgenol. *102:* 587 (1968).

10. WANG, C. C. and SCHULZ, M. D.: The role of radiation therapy in the management of carcinoma of the sigmoid, rectosigmoid, and rectum. Radiology *79:* 1 (1962).

Author's address: Dr. CLIFFORD V. ALLEN, Department of Radiation Therapy, University of Oregon Medical School, 3181 S. W. Sam Jackson Park Road, *Portland, OR 97201* (USA).

Front. Radiation Ther. Onc., vol. 5, pp. 163–176
(Karger, Basel/München/Paris/New York 1970)

Preoperative Radiation Therapy
for Carcinoma of the Lung:
Report of a National VA Controlled Study[1]

B. ROSWIT, G. A. HIGGINS, W. SHIELDS and R. J. KEEHN

Department of Medicine and Surgery and US Veterans Administration, Surgical Adjuvant
Cancer Chemotherapy Group, Bronx, N.Y.

Introduction

The present outlook for cure for most patients with lung cancer remains grim. The mortality in this country alone is expected to increase from the present rate of over 50,000 deaths per year to more than 85,000 by 1980. The US Veterans Administration, with more than 100,000 adult male hospital patients, has assumed a responsible and major role in the search for a better means to treat the operable and inoperable patient. Prospective protocols, national in scope, involving more than 6000 subjects, have been in progress since 1957 – investigating chemotherapy, radiotherapy and surgery in the management of this formidable disease [6, 7 8, 14, 15, 17, 18, 19].

In this paper we wish to present a preliminary report on the outcome of a controlled study of the effect on survival of preoperative radiation therapy (4000–5000 rads in 4–6 weeks), employing high energy beams in clinically operable male patients with histologically proven carcinoma of the lung.

Basis for Study

There is already well-documented experimental radiobiological data to suggest that preoperative irradiation, for subjects with operable cancer, may improve operability and resectability and reduce the chance for local recurrences and distant metastasis [11].

Thus the probability for cure may be enhanced. Clinical trials in lung cancer which appear to support these premises have been carried out in this country and abroad in the past decade by Bromley and Szur [4], Bloedorn and Cowley [2, 3], Paulson [10] and others [1, 9].

Particularly impressive is the evidence that the primary lesion and even the regional nodes could be sterilized in one-third to one-half the cases. Survival rates are described as an improvement over what might be expected without preoperative irradiation.

In none of these studies were controls and randomization employed, so that a valid comparison could be made between irradiated and non-irradiated patients. To make this test, we initiated a national prospective protocol in December 1962 in 25 of our major VA hospitals in 18 States, with statistical support from the Follow-up Agency of the National Research Council.

Method

The criteria for admission to the study included male patients with clinically operable and histologically proven carcinoma of the bronchus, with no evidence of distant metastasis, medically acceptable for surgery, without previous operation for the same lung tumor, and without other tumors or previous anti-cancer therapy.

To date, a total of 339 patients have been admitted to the study and randomized to (1) preoperative radiation followed by thoracotomy in 4–6 weeks and (2) surgery alone. Treatment was assigned randomly by the British envelope system. As in all other VA protocols, we compared the proportion of patients in each group surviving to a given day. In our experience, this method, compared to long-range survival data, has proved to be the most reliable index for prompt and reproducible comparison of different therapeutic regimens.

In the preoperative irradiation program, our objective was to treat both the primary lesion and mediastinum with the best possible dose distribution within the treatment volume. After treatment, the patient was re-evaluated for thoracotomy and operated if there were no contraindications.

In the treatment planning and delivery, modern technology was used to maximum advantage and a high standard of quality was achieved. High energy photon beams were employed, including Cobalt-60, 1 MeV and 2 MeV generators and 6 MeV linear accelerators. Treatment plans, technical data, and calculations were carefully reviewed by the Chairman of the Radiation Group and Consulting Medical Physicist to ensure conformity with protocol standards. Field arrangements were employed according to the judgement of collaborating radiologists and physicists. Parallel opposing fields were recommended, and were employed in the majority of cases. A moderate dose-time fractionation system (1000 rads per 5 day week) was adopted to minimize the risk of severe radiation injury which might delay, complicate or even prohibit surgery. Overall treatment time was planned for 4 weeks (minimum) to 6 weeks (maximum) and a tumor dose of 4000–5000 rads.

Operation was performed as soon as possible after randomization, usually within 2 weeks. The type of operation – exploratory, lobectomy or pneumonectomy – was left to the decision of the individual surgeon. No effort was made to standardize operative principles. The resection was considered *curative* if pathologic study showed no tumor left behind; *palliative* if tumor was found at the cut margins of the specimen or in biopsies obtained from residual tissue left in the thorax at operation.

Results

Eligibility. A total of 339 were accepted into the study, but 8 were excluded because of violation of requirements for eligibility. Of these, 4 were in the treated group (preoperative X-ray) and 4 in the controls (operation only) leaving for final evaluation 166 treated patients and 165 controls, for a total of 331 cases.

Composition. The two groups, treated and controls, were scanned for significant differences in important characteristics which might influence treatment evaluation. Similar distributions were found in all but one of these characteristics. They include age, race, tumor type, previous cancer therapy, physical evidence of cancer, other pulmonary disease, significant non-pulmonary disease, duration of symptoms and smoking history. Of particular interest is the fact that there were only 7 non-smokers (2.1%) in the entire group of 331 patients. The treated group included a higher proportion of patients under 60 years of age than the controls, 52 and 39% respectively.

Radiation therapy. A total of 157 patients received preoperative irradiation from 3000 to 6000 rads. Nine patients were never started (for medical reasons) but were not excluded from the analysis of the group to avoid bias in the comparison of treatment.

About 50% of the patients received 4000–4999 rads. The lower dose level (below 4000 rads) was given to 27 patients (17.2%) because of intercurrent illness, appearance of distant metastasis, refusal of further treatment or death of the patient. The high-dose regimen (above 5000 rads) was delivered to 48 patients (30.6%) early in the study by a limited number of our colleagues who were impressed with the apparent symptomatic and/or radiographic evidence of improvement. Only 3 patients had a minimum dose in excess of 6000 rads. Treatment plans and dose calculations were carefully re-examined and found to reflect a generally high quality of performance.

Surgical therapy. The *operability rate* was far better in the controls (93%) than in the X-ray group (64%). Fully 36% of the irradiated patients never came to surgery because of death, refusal of operation or intercurrent medical problems (table I, II). Nor was the *resectability rate* improved by preoperative X-ray treatment. Approximately 50% in each group underwent resections.

Table I. Surgical treatment

	No. op.	Thoracot.	Resection
X-ray (166)	60	20	86
	36.1%	12.0%	51.8%
Controls (165)	12	63	90
	7.3%	38.2%	54.5%

Table II. Inoperable group – no surgery

	X-ray	Control
No surgery, *total*	60	12
Inoperable cancer	22	3
Inoperable (not cancer)	10	5
Refused surgery	13	3
Died before surgery	14	1
Unknown	1	0

Operation was promptly performed after randomization in the control group (76% within 10 days, table III). In the X-ray treated group operation was not performed until 50 days or longer after randomization in 60% of the patients. In 46% of these subjects there was a delay of 10 weeks or more before surgery was feasible.

Pneumonectomy, with extra-pulmonary dissection, was the most common procedure in both groups undergoing resection. Only 12% in each group had lobectomies. The majority of resected patients in each group had *curative* operations. No apparent tumor was left behind in 85% of the X-ray group and in 91% of the controls.

Complete sterilization of the cancer was accomplished by irradiation in 27% (23 cases), while cancer was described in all of the resected specimens in the operation-only group, and in these patients there were more squamous cell and undifferentiated lesions.

Complications. There was no significant difference in the percentage or type of postoperative complications in either group, X-ray treated or control (table IV). There were slightly but not significantly more cardiovascular complications in the irradiated patients.

Table III. Interval between randomization and operation

Days, random. to op.	X-ray		Control	
	Number	Percent	Number	Percent
Total cases	166	100	165	100.0
No operation	60	36.1	12	7.3
0–9 days	2	1.2	126	76.4
10–29 days	0	0.0	25	15.2
30–49 days	4	2.4	1	0.6
50–69 days	23	13.9	1	0.6
70–89 days	48	28.9	0	0.0
90 days	26	15.7	0	0.0
110 days or more	3	1.8	0	0.0

Table IV. Postoperative complications

Complication	X-ray		Control		P
	Number	Percent	Number	Percent	
Resected cases, total	85	100.0	90	100.0	
Patients with complications[1]					
Technical	15	17.6	14	15.6	>0.9
Pulmonary	15	17.6	14	15.6	>0.9
Cardiovascular	18	21.2	13	14.4	0.33
Hematologic	3	3.5	2	2.2	>0.9
Thromboembolic	2	2.4	2	2.2	>0.9
Septic	2	2.4	2	2.2	>0.9

[1] Each reported complication type has been counted, regardless of whether or not other types were reported for the same patient.

However, the increased morbidity did not have much influence on the 30 day postoperative mortality (table V). The mortality in the resected patients was approximately 12% in both groups.

Table V. Thirty-day surgical mortality

| Operation | X-ray 30-day deaths | | | Control 30-day deaths | | | P |
	Cases	Number	Percent	Cases	Number	Percent	
All operations	106	13	12.3	153	24	15.7	0.55
Thoracotomy only	20	2	10.0	63	13	20.6	>0.9
Resected	86	11	12.8	90	11	12.2	>0.9

In the X-ray treated group there was little acute morbidity directly attributable to the irradiation such as skin reactions, radiation sickness, marrow depression or acute pneumonitis. These will be reviewed in another report.

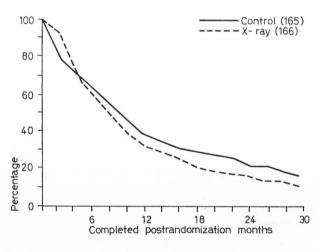

Fig. 1. Survival from randomization, all patients.

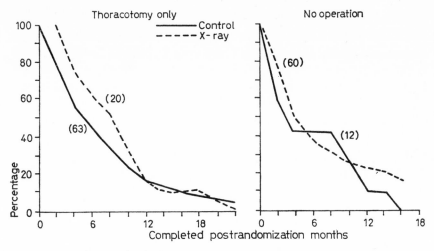

Fig. 2. Survival from randomization.

Survival. When the survival of *all* patients admitted to the study are compared from the time of *randomization,* there is no statistically significant difference between the preoperative X-ray group and the operation-only group (fig. 1). Nor is there any such difference when one considers only patients who had no operation, or even in those who had only a thoracotomy (fig. 2). In the latter, there is an early displacement of the curve due to deferment of surgery in the X-ray treated group.

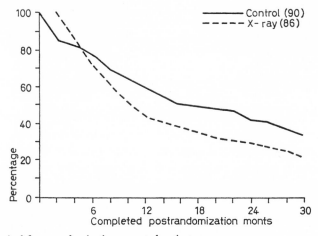

Fig. 3. Survival from randomization, resected patients.

However, a major difference is apparent when we compare the survival of *resected* cases from the time of randomization (fig. 3). Combined therapy in resected cases does appear to have a harmful effect on the survival of these patients. The survival at 12 months is only 44% when compared with that for the promptly resected control group (60%) (P<0.05).

This deleterious influence of combined treatment on survival is more strikingly demonstrated when we compare survival curves of *resected* patients in both groups (treated and controls) from the *time of operation* (fig. 4).

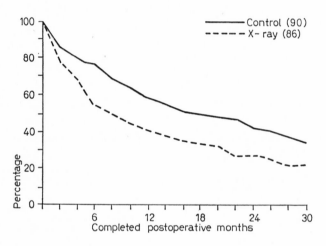

Fig. 4. Survival from operation, resected patients.

When the first 18 postoperative months were separated into successive 3-month intervals and the groups compared, the survival difference was found concentrated in the first 6 postoperative months. At 6-months the survival is shown to be 55% for treated patients, compared with 77% for the controls (significant at the one percent level). This effect of irradiation is even more pronounced when we compared the *curative resection* group – treated versus controls – at the 6-month level (table VI).

Table VI. Six month postoperative survival

Resectability and clinical impression	Treated			Control			
	Total cases	Survival Number	Percent	Total cases	Survival Number	Percent	P
Total	106	55	51.9	153	94	61.4	>0.16
Resectable	86	47	54.7	90	69	76.7	0.004
Curative	74	41	55.4	71	58	81.7	0.001
Other	12	6	50.0	19	11	57.9	>0.9
Thoracotomy	20	8	40.0	63	25	39.7	>0.9

Despite the fact that no demonstrable tumor was found in the resected specimens of 23 patients in the irradiated group, this did not appear to have much influence on their longevity, when compared with control patients with cancer in the specimen (fig. 6). Beyond eight months postoperative their outlook is somewhat better than for X-ray cases with residual tumor, but not yet as good as in the controls (fig. 6).

Of the 23 patients with negative resected specimens, 16 have already died. The post-mortems in 10 of these subjects showed tumor in 6, and in 2 of these there was disease in the operative site. Of the remaining 6 deceased patients, 4 were not autopsied but death was ascribed to recurrent and/or metastatic cancer on clinical evidence.

Discussion

We have conducted an interdisciplinary randomized VA study with effective controls, involving 331 patients with operable lung cancer and have failed to demonstrate improvement in survival through preoperative high energy radiation therapy in dose levels from 3000 to 6000 rads. In fact, when these two major stresses on the lung cancer patient are combined (high energy radiation plus pneumonectomy) there seems to be a deleterious effect on the longevity of resected patients, concentrated in the first six postoperative months. This influence was not noted in irradiated patients who underwent thoracotomy only or had no surgery at all.

We have critically reviewed our data to find a reasonable and acceptable explanation for this unhappy outcome. The characteristics of the two groups were re-examined for significant *differences* in *composition* and none were found. They included age at surgery, duration of symptoms, smoking history, other pulmonary diseases, other significant non-pulmonary diseases, year of surgery, operation performed, site of resection and biopsy diagnosis before randomization and after resection.

Next, we assessed the influence of *lymph node involvement* in the resected specimen (fig. 5). The finding of positive nodes did predict poor survival. The presence or absence of tumor in lymph nodes, however, appeared to be unrelated to the poorer survival following resection seen in X-ray treated cases.

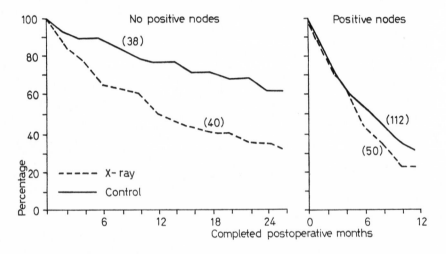

Fig. 5. Survival from operation.

The *sterilization of the primary cancer* and/or involved regional lymph nodes would seem to be a good omen for survival, but we have no such evidence in our own data (fig. 6). We find support for this finding in the pilot study of Bromley and Szur in England [4] who sterilized fully 37% of the lesions in 66 patients. Only 6 of these 24 patients were alive at 2 to 5 years after the combined procedure. Baker, Cowley and Lindberg at the University of Maryland provide further documentation in their follow-up of Bloedorn's patients 'locally cured' by preoperative irradiation at radical dose levels. Of 17 patients so 'cured' only one was alive (3½ years) at the time of the report [1]. They conclude that, in their selected study, complete control of local disease was, in itself, rarely sufficient to extend long-term survival.

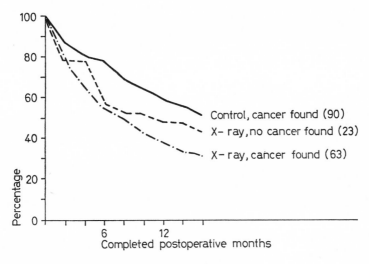

Fig. 6. Survival from operation.

An outstanding difference between the two groups is the very considerable *delay in resection* of the cancer because of the X-ray therapy. Over 60% of irradiated patients had a delay of 50 to 110 days between randomization and operation. Clearly, delay is a factor in the final outcome. We note its influence (table VII) when we compare survival at 6 months after curative resection in relation to delay of operation. However, the difference in survival rates in the treated and control groups did not occur in patients who did not have any lung tumor removed, in spite of the delay. Surely, some difference should be anticipated if the delay factor was of major importance.

Finally, if the impact of *irradiation* is a major factor in the poorer survival of resected patients, this should be a dose-related phenomenon – and indeed it appears to be. There is a decrease in survival with increasing dose (table VII). A higher dose of preoperative X-ray therapy appears to be more closely related to impaired longevity than is the delay period before definitive surgery, but the evidence is not yet conclusive.

Table VII. Survival six months after curative resection by delay of operation and X-ray dose

Minimum tumor dose (r)	Under 80 days			80 days or more		
		Six month survival			Six month survival	
	Cases	Number	Percent	Cases	Number	Percent
Total	31	20	64.5	43	21	48.8
Under 4000 rads	3	3	100.0	2	2	100.0
4000–4999 rads	22	15	68.2	21	11	52.4
5000 rads and over	6	2	33.3	18	7	38.9
Unknown	—	—	—	2	1	50.0

It may be that radiation injury to the lungs, heart and mediastinum is too large a burden for the patient who is undergoing major pulmonary resection, which further reduces his cardiopulmonary reserve and potential for survival. This burden seems to be displayed to his disadvantage in the first six postoperative months, the period of concentrated mortality in this group of patients. After this period, the survival curves of irradiated and non-irradiated resected patients appear to run parallel. Clinical and autopsy data are being studied to define the principal and contributory causes of death and these will be reported later. Nearly all deceased patients appear to die *with* cancer, local and/or metastatic. We must conclude that *routine* preoperative radiation for patients with clinically operable bronchogenic carcinoma, as employed in this protocol, offers no benefit over surgery alone.

A collaborative study of a similar nature undertaken by 17 cooperating Medical Centers, under the aegis of the Committee on Radiation Therapy Studies recently reported no gain in longevity through preoperative irradiation [5]. It is of keen interest that their survival curves, including all cases from the date of randomization, match ours (fig. 1) to a remarkable degree.

On the basis of our own findings, we are no longer entering VA patients into our preoperative irradiation protocol, but will continue to study the incoming data on surviving cases and will report the outcome in a later communication.

Acknowledgements

This study was conducted at 25 Veterans Administration Hospitals under the auspices of the Departments of Medicine and Surgery. The *Coordinator* was Dr. LYNDON E. LEE, Jr.; the *Surgical Chairman* – Dr. GEORGE HIGGINS; *Radiation Chairman* – Dr. BERNARD ROSWIT; *Consulting Physicist* – Mr. CYPRIAN B. REID; *Statistician* – Mr. ROBERT J. KEEHN of the Follow-up Agency, National Research Council. *Veterans Administration Hospitals* in the following cities and the following surgical collaborators participated in this study: Boston, MA, RICHARD W. DWIGHT; Bronx, NY, PHILIP COOPER; Brooklyn, NY, HARRY H. LeVEEN; Chicago, IL (Res.), THOMAS W. SHIELDS; Cincinnati, OH, CARL G. SCHOWENGERDT; Cleveland, OH, JERRY S. WOLKOFF; Dallas, TX, ROBERT HAYS; East Orange, NJ, OSCAR SERLIN; Hines, IL, WILLIAM S. WALSH; Houston, TX, PAUL JORDAN; Iowa City, IA, RICHARD LAWTON; Jackson, MS, J. HAROLD CONN; Kansas City, MO, ALFRED HEILBRUNN; Long Beach, CA, GEORGE L. JULER; Memphis, TN, FELIX HUGHES; Minneapolis, MN, EDWARD HUMPHREY; Martinez, CA, JOHN V. SMITH; Philadelphia, PA, STANLEY J. DUDRICK; Pittsburgh, PA, FRANCIS JACKSON; Providence, RI, H. W. HARROWER; San Juan, PR, JOSE H. AMADEO; St. Louis, MO, ROBERT C. DONALDSON; Syracuse, NY, LLOYD S. ROGERS; Washington, DC, GEORGE A. HIGGINS; Wood, WI, GALE L. MENDELOFF.

We are especially grateful to our VA radiological colleagues who contributed their effort and their skill to the conduct of this national study.

Summary

(1) The United States Veterans Administration has assumed a major and responsible role in the search for better means to improve the outlook for patients with lung cancer through the conduct of several national protocols assessing the role of surgery, radiation and chemicals. (2) In this randomized VA Lung Cancer Study, we have found that high energy preoperative irradiation (3000–6000 rads) has not improved survival in 339 male patients with clinically operable, histologically verified lung cancer. (3) When all cases are analyzed from the time of randomization, there appears to be a harmful influence on the longevity of those patients who are fully resected after irradiation. This influence is concentrated in the first six postoperative months.

References

1. BAKER, N. H., COWLEY, R. A. and LINBERG, E.: A Follow-up in patients with bronchogenic carcinoma 'locally cured' by preoperative irradiation. J. thorac. cardiovasc. Surg. *46:* 298–309 (1963).
2. BLOEDORN, F. and COWLEY, A.: Preoperative irradiation in bronchogenic carcinoma. Amer. J. Roentgenol. *92:* 77 (1964).

3. BLOEDORN, F. G.: Rationale and benefit of preoperative irradiation in lung cancer.
   J. amer. med. Ass. *196:* 340–341 (1966).
4. BROMLEY, L. L. and SZUR, L.: Combined radiotherapy and resection for carcinoma of
   the bronchus: Experiences with 66 patients. Lancet *ii:* 937–941 (1955).
5. Committee for Radiation Therapy Studies: Preoperative irradiation of cancer of the
   lung: Preliminary report of a therapeutic trial. Cancer, vol. 23, p. 419–429 (1969).
6. HIGGINS, G. A.: Preoperative irradiation for lung carcinoma: The VA National Study.
   Symposium on Cancer Therapy by Integrated Radiation and Operation (Thomas,
   Springfield, 1970).
7. HUGHES, F. A. and HIGGINS, G. A.: Veterans administration surgical adjuvant lung
   cancer chemotherapy study: Present status. J. thorac. Surg. *44:* 295–304 (1962).
8. HUGHES, F. A.; HIGGINS, G. and BEEBE, G. W.: Present status of surgical adjuvant
   lung chemotherapy. J. amer. med. Ass. *196:* 343–344 (1966).
9. MERCADO, C. A.; WIZENBERG, M. J. and LINBERG, E. J.: Preoperative Irradiation in
   Bronchogenic Carcinoma. Amer. J. Roentgenol. *92:* 77–87 (1964).
10. PAULSON, D. L.: The survival rate in superior sulcus tumors treated by presurgical
    irradiation. J. amer. med. Ass. *196:* 342 (1966).
11. POWERS, W. E. and TOLMACH, L. J.: Preoperative radiation therapy: Biological basis
    and experimental investigations. Nature *83:* 509–519 (1964).
12. ROSWIT, B.: Radiation therapy and radioisotopes; in SPAIN Diagnosis and treatment of
    tumors of the chest, chapter 20, pp. 299–334 (Grune & Stratton, New York 1960).
13. ROSWIT, B.: Bronchogenic carcinoma, stages 3 and 4. Palliation by chemotherapy.
    J. amer. med. Ass. *196:* 848–849 (1966).
14. ROSWIT, B.; PATNO, M. E.; RAPP, R.; VEINBERGS, A.; FEDER, B.; STUHLBARG, J. and
    REID, C. B.: The survival of patients with inoperable lung cancer: A large-scale ran-
    domized study of radiation therapy versus placebo. Radiology, *90:* 688–697 (1968)
15. ROSWIT, B.: Outlook for patients with lung cancer, Hospital Practice *3:* 22–27 (1968).
16. RUBIN, P.: Comment: Combination therapy-irradiation, surgery and chemotherapy.
    J. amer. med. Ass. *196:* 348 (1966).
17. SHIELDS, T. W.; HIGGINS, G. A.; LAWTON, R.; HEILBRUNN, A.; KEEHN, R. J. and
    ROSWIT, B.: Preoperative X-ray therapy as an adjuvant in the treatment of broncho-
    genic carcinoma. J. thorac. cardiovasc. Surgery (accepted for publication).
18. Veterans Administration Adjuvant Cancer Chemotherapy Cooperative Group: Evalua-
    tion of chemotherapeutic agents as adjuvants to surgery in twenty-two veterans admi-
    nistration hospitals: Experimental design. Cancer Chemother. Rep. *20:* 81–97 (1962).
19. WOLF, J.; PATNO, M. E.; ROSWIT, B. and D'ESOPO, N.: Controlled study of survival
    of patients with clinically inoperable lung cancer treated with radiation therapy. Amer.
    J. med. *40:* 360–367 (1966).

Author's address: Dr. BERNARD ROSWIT, US Veterans Administration Hospital, 130 West
Kingsbridge Rd., *Bronx, NY 10468* (USA).

Front. Radiation Ther. Onc., vol. 5, pp. 177–187
(Karger, Basel/München/Paris/New York 1970)

The Role of Preoperative Radiation Therapy in the Surgical Management of Carcinoma in the Superior Pulmonary Sulcus

DONALD L. PAULSON[1]

Bronchogenic carcinomas developed peripherally in the apex of the lung and invading the superior pulmonary sulcus (Pancoast tumors) are frequently low grade epidermoid carcinomas which grow slowly and metastasize late. Situated in the narrow confines of the apex of the chest, they invade the lymphatics in the endothoracic fascia and involve, by direct extension, the lower roots of the brachial plexus, the intercostal nerves, the stellate ganglion, the sympathetic chain, adjacent ribs and vertebrae, producing severe pain and the Horner's syndrome. In the past, lesions in this location have been generally considered as inaccessible to complete resection and resistant to radiation therapy. Previous experience indicates that average expected time of survival after diagnosis, reported in the literature and in our own experience, has been 10 to 14 months. In a series of 23 patients previously observed, the longest survival after diagnosis of 15 patients receiving no specific treatment or irradiation alone was 10 to 13 months. Only 3 of 8 patients treated by resection followed by irradiation survived more than 1 year, the longest survival being 27 months.

From 1956 through 1968, 45 patients with carcinomas in the superior pulmonary sulcus have been treated by combined preoperative irradiation and resection (table I). In addition during the same period, 12 patients were considered inoperable at time of

---

[1] Chief, Thoracic Surgical Section, Baylor University Medical Center and Clinical Professor of Thoracic and Cardiovascular Surgery, The University of Texas (Southwestern) Medical School.

diagnosis, 8 patients became inoperable due to metastases during the interval prior to surgery, 3 patients refused surgery and 1 proved to be non-resectable at operation. There were 2 operative mortalities. Of the remaining 43 patients who survived combined presurgical irradiation and extended resection, 10 of 30 patients eligible have survived 5 years, including 5 for 10 years (fig. 1).

Table I. Carcinoma in the superior sulcus, preoperative irradiation and extended resection, 1956–1968

	No. of patients
Completed combined treatment	45
Inoperable originally	12
Became inoperable	8
Non-resectable	1
Refused surgery	3
Total	69

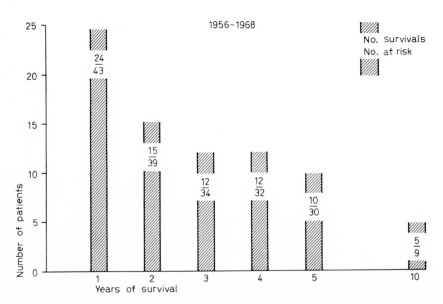

Fig. 1. Survival after combined irradiation and resection for carcinoma in the superior pulmonary sulcus. Twelve patients have survived 3 years, after which there have been no deaths due to bronchogenic carcinoma.

There have been no deaths due to carcinoma after 3 years, at which period 12 patients have survived and are well. Calculated by the life table method, there has been a 38% survival at 2 years and 33% at 5 years. Although previous experience does not constitute a strict control, the results of preoperative irradiation for superior sulcus tumors over a 10-year period would appear to be significant in the conversion of a hopeless lesion in this location to a resectable one in 80% of the patients, with prolonged survival in 33% of those who completed the combined treatment.

Two of 3 patients who refused surgery died within a year and the third has survived over 5 years following radiation therapy alone (unproved by tissue diagnosis).

Rationale of Treatment

In this series, a histologic diagnosis has not been obtained prior to the institution of combined treatment for bronchogenic carcinoma in the superior sulcus. It is believed that in general the inaccessibility of the lesion, the risk of dissemination, and increased morbidity through surgical interference, together with the adverse effect of biopsy on radiosensitivity of the tumor, contraindicate exploration for this purpose. Interference or violation of the vascular bed of the tumor and its lymphatics, or the introduction of hematoma, low grade infection or inflammation, may lower the oxygen tension and decrease its sensitivity to irradiation, thus jeopardizing the opportunity for cure. Tissue proof is simply deferred to the time of resection, 4–6 weeks later.

The clinical syndrome of severe pain in the shoulder and along the ulnar distribution in the arm (due to involvement of nerve roots C8 and T1), together with roentgenographic evidence of a tumor in the apex of the chest, with or without bone destruction and a Horner's syndrome, is diagnostic of a neoplastic process in the superior pulmonary sulcus invading the chest wall (fig. 2). Other lesions, including metastatic neoplasms or inflammatory lesions such as fibrosing pneumonitis or tuberculosis, may be confusing, but the severity and location of the pain, the radiologic appearance and statistical preponderance today emphasize the probability of bronchogenic carcinoma as a cause.

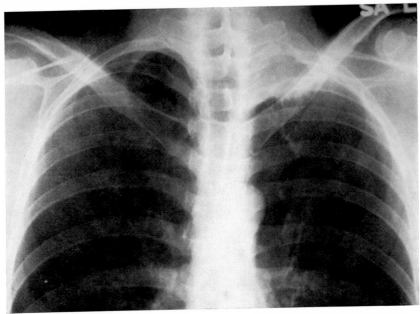

Fig. 2. Roentgenogram illustrating a tumor mass in the left apex of the chest with destruction of the second rib.

Errors in diagnosis occurred in 5 patients treated by means of preoperative irradiation. Tuberculosis constituted the most common error, being found in 3 patients. When the clinical syndrome is atypical and the diagnosis doubtful, a calculated risk is taken and antimicrobial therapy as well as irradiation are instituted in preparation for a thoracotomy. Open biopsy of the cupola of the pleura through a supraclavicular scalenotomy incision or needle biopsy are useful procedures for inoperable or doubtful cases.

The purpose of presurgical irradiation is to modify the extent of the disease so that the lesion is better localized and thus more completely resectable with improved results, but without increased morbidity. The tumor dose used for bronchogenic carcinoma in the superior pulmonary sulcus is 3000 R given in 10 treatments over 12 elapsed days. It is approximately 75% of the cancerocidal dose of 4200 R delivered in 2 weeks' time based on the Strandquist curve for squamous cell carcinoma of the skin. The aim of the subcancerocidal dose is to localize the lesion and inhibit dissemination or implantation by destruction of the tumor cells at the periphery, to produce sclerosis of the vascular bed and the lymphatics, and damage to the viability and reproductive integrity of malignant cells not resected, implanted or disseminated at the time of operation. Full cancerocidal dosage carries the risk of increased radiologic and operative morbidity by sterilization or depopulation of normal tissue cells necessary for repair. The radiation-operative interval has been shortened from the original 4–6 weeks to 3–4 weeks.

Although the optimum dosage and interval between radiation and surgery remains to be determined, clinical and experimental observations indicate that presurgical irradiation in doses that are not sufficient to completely sterilize or cause regression of the tumors treated, decreases local recurrence, prevents the growth of tumor cells after dissemination and increases survival when compared with irradiation or surgery alone [1, 2, 3, 4, 5, 7].

Pain is frequently improved or palliated by irradiation although it frequently recurs and shows no correlation with prognosis. Destroyed ribs may be reconstituted as a result of irradiation. Three of 10 5-year survivors had definite bone involvement including ribs and vertebrae. The mass of the lesion may not necessarily diminish as a result of the irradiation due to replacement by scar and non-neoplastic tissue. There has been no increase in morbidity attributable to radiation therapy in the dosage range recommended. One patient who received 4500 R as preoperative therapy elsewhere has developed a radiation neuritis.

The surgical technique for resection of a superior sulcus tumor is an extended *en bloc* resection of the chest wall usually including posterior portions of the first 3 ribs, their transverse processes, portions of the upper thoracic vertebrae, the intercostal nerves, the lower trunk of the brachial plexus, the stellate ganglion and the upper fibers of the sympathetic chain together with the involved lung, resected either by means of lobectomy or segmental resection [6].

Pathology

Resection 3–6 weeks after the completion of radiation therapy has established the histologic diagnosis of bronchogenic carcinoma in all cases included in this series except for the second patient, now surviving 12 years, who presented a classical Pancoast syndrome and in whom irradiation is believed to have completely sterilized the tumor. Pathologic examination of resected specimens from all other patients has shown a profound alteration in the neoplasm. Grossly, there is a peripheral pseudo-capsule and central degeneration. The periphery of the tumor has been reduced to an amorphous mass so that it is necessary to take sections deep within the lesion to find typical neoplastic cells. In the intermediate zone, scattered cells with pyknotic nuclei can be seen as remains of damaged cancer cells. Pathologic findings indicate marked destruction, degeneration, giant cell formation, fibrosis and localization of the neoplastic mass by irradiation so that it is possible to carry the line of resection much closer to the lesion without fear of dissemination or subsequent local recurrence.

Cell type was identifiable in 44 of 45 lesions resected after irradiation. There were 21 squamous cell carcinomas, 17 undifferentiated large cell carcinomas, 6 adenocarcinomas and 1 undetermined cell type (table II). Of the patients surviving 3 or more years, 7 had squamous cell carcinomas, 3 undifferentiated large cell carcinomas, 1 adenocarcinoma, and in 1 the cell type was undetermined.

Table II. Tumor pathology in 45 patients (1956–1968) completing preoperative irradiation and resection for carcinoma in the superior pulmonary sulcus

Cell type	Number	3-year survivors
Squamous cell	21	7
Large cell undifferentiated	17	3
Adenocarcinoma	6	1
Undetermined	1	1
Total	45	12

Discussion

Bronchogenic carcinomas in the superior pulmonary sulcus produce a characteristic clinical syndrome described by Pancoast. In the past, lesions in this location have been generally considered as hopeless from the standpoint of therapy either by irradiation or complete resection. The results of presurgical irradiation for lesions in this location over a 10-year period would appear to be significant in that resection was possible in 80% of the patients followed by prolonged survival in 33% of those who completed the combined treatment.

Carcinomas in the superior pulmonary sulcus are usually either well differentiated epidermoid carcinomas or of the large cell undifferentiated type. Whereas they are locally invasive of the surrounding structures in the narrow confines of the apex of the chest, they frequently do not metastasize distantly until late and they are radiosensitive. Complete sterilization by irradiation is possible and may have been accomplished in the second patient in the series as well as one patient who refused surgery (unproved by tissue diagnosis) and has survived over 5 years. On the other hand, 44 of 45 resected specimens after irradiation contained identifiable and presumably viable carcinoma. Although an occasional long-term survivor following irradiation alone has been reported, the results do not approach a 30% rate. Similarly, radical resection with or without the use of radon seeds or postoperative irradiation may lead to an occasional prolonged survival.

It is believed that complete resection without preoperative irradiation is usually impossible for superior sulcus tumors which frequently involve adjacent ribs, vertebrae, nerve trunks and lymphatics in both the perineural sheaths and the endothoracic fascia. In fact, in most cases the bulk of the tumor is found to be extrapulmonary. The extrapulmonary extensions of the carcinoma make the lesion incompletely resectable. If not too extensive, these appear to respond to irradiation, thus improving the possibility of complete removal. In addition, tumor cells at the periphery are destroyed and a pseudo-capsule composed of an amorphous mass of fibrous tissue results from the irradiation, thus lessening the likelihood of implantation or dissemination.

Objection may be made to the use of irradiation based on a clinical diagnosis alone without tissue proof of the carcinoma. Admittedly errors may be made, but it is believed that the characteristic syndrome of a carcinoma in the superior pulmonary sulcus can be diagnosed clinically with better than 90% accuracy. Where there is reason to doubt the diagnosis, a calculated risk may be taken and antimicrobial therapy instituted along with the irradiation, since tuberculosis constitutes the most likely cause for error. Should histologic diagnosis be insisted upon or desirable as in inoperable or doubtful cases, needle biopsy or open biopsy of the cupola through a scalenotomy incision may be employed. The inaccessibility of most of these lesions, the risks of implantation or dissemination and the adverse effects on radiosensitivity by operative interference all mitigate against insistence on exploration for tissue proof prior to irradiation. In reality the timing of histologic diagnosis is simply deferred since it is obtained at the time of resection in operable cases.

Summary

Preoperative irradiation has been used in 57 patients with bronchogenic carcinoma in the superior pulmonary sulcus from 1956 through 1968. Eight patients became inoperable during the interval prior to surgery, 3 patients refused surgery and 1 proved to be non-resectable at the time of operation. Resection was completed in 45 patients, and there were 2 operative mortalities.

Of 43 patients who survived combined presurgical irradiation and extended resection, 10 of 30 patients eligible have survived over 5 years, including 5 for 10 years. Calculated by the life table method, there has been a 38% survival at 2 years and 33% at 5 years.

The rationale of treatment is based on omission of a tissue diagnosis prior to the institution of radiation therapy in moderate subcancerocidal dosage followed by extended *en bloc* resection of the lesion.

References

1. Henschke, U. K.; Frazell, E. L.; Basaris, B. S.; Nickson, J. J.; Tollefsen, H. R. and Strong, E. W.: Local recurrences after radical neck dissection with or without preoperative X-ray therapy. Radiology *82:* 331 (1964).
2. Hoye, R. C. and Smith, R. R.: Effectiveness of small amounts of preoperative irradiation in preventing growth of tumor cells disseminated at surgery: Experimental study. Cancer *14:* 284 (1963).
3. Inch, W. R. and McCredie, J. A.: Effect of small dose of X-radiation on local recurrence of tumors in rats and mice. Cancer *16:* 595 (1963).
4. Inch, W. R. and McCredie, J. A.: Preoperative use of a single dose of X-rays: Local cancer recurrence. Arch. Surg., Chicago *89:* 398 (1964).
5. Powers, W. E. and Palmer, L. A.: Biologic basis of preoperative radiation treatment. Amer. J. Roentgenol. *102:* 176 (1968).
6. Shaw, R. R.; Paulson, D. L. and Kee, J. L., Jr.: Treatment of the superior sulcus tumor by irradiation followed by resection. Ann. Surg. *154:* 29 (1961).
7. Stearns, M. D., Jr.; Berg, J. W. and Deddish, M. A.: Preoperative irradiation of cancer of the rectum. Dis. Colon. Rect. *4:* 403 (1961).

Author's address: Dr. Donald L. Paulson, 3810 Swiss Avenue, *Dallas, TX 75204* (USA).

Discussion

Moderator:

MILTON J. PEARL, M. D., Associate Chief of Surgery and Chairman, Cancer Committee, Mt. Zion Hospital and Medical Center, *San Francisco, Calif.*

Discussant:

H. BRODIE STEPHENS, M. D., Clinical Professor of Surgery (Emeritus); Chief of Staff, University of California Medical Center, *San Francisco, Calif.*

STEPHENS: We are greatly indebted to Dr. DOGGETT for this very careful study of a good many cases of squamous cell carcinoma of the esophagus. This subject was reviewed by CADE in 1963, and of about 119 cases surgically treated only 2 survived for 5 years, so that Dr. DOGGETT need not apologize for combined therapy. As Dr. PAULSON has done, one should select cases preoperatively and understand that these are going to be the favorable ones. Dr. ALLEN (on cancer of the rectum) and Dr. PAULSON (on cancer of lung superior sulcus) have definitely demonstrated that there are improved results by combined treatment. Dr. ALLEN, is it necessary to explore the patient? If a patient has a carcinoma of the rectosigmoid and at the proctoscopic examination, he has cardiovascular complication, why not give him radiation therapy as you have outlined and then operate on him? I think the fact that you demonstrated that 9 out of 18 patients that were inoperable because of fixation became resectable is significant.

ALLEN: When we began this study, there were at least 2 standard references on preoperative radiation therapy that said if radiation therapy is to be given preoperatively to the colon, a colostomy is mandatory, and it was for that reason that we did the routine colostomies. We are now doing exactly as you have suggested and no longer do colostomies routinely. Palliative therapy is worthwhile in cases with obstructions when there are known metastases. We are accumulating a series of these cases.

PEARL: It's a known surgical fact that when patients with carcinoma of the colon are operated on with antibiotic preparation and the colon is sterilized, the incidence of local recurrence is much higher. This has been attributed to the fact that the bacteria probably keep the cancer cells from implanting at the suture line, but it might be that there's more to it than that, particularly in view of Dr. ALLEN's improved survival data related to colostomies.

ROSWIT: I was impressed 5 years ago with a retrospective study at Memorial that showed a very distinctive difference between patients with cancer of the rectum who received preoperative irradiation, 1,500 rads, conventional medium volt therapy, to the whole lower abdomen and pelvis as compared to those that were not irradiated. In one group with involved nodes, there were 37% 5 year survivals in the preoperative irradiated patients as against 23% for those not irradiated. In 10 years a nearly 3 times better prognosis. It seemed to me that here again, a test had to be made of this premise in a prospective study. Twenty-three of our Veterans Administration hospitals, of 500 to 1,000 beds, have an incidence of 2,000 cancers of the rectum each year. Our cases were properly randomized and we treated 305 cases; this time not with conventional medium volt therapy, but with cobalt and high energy radiations, as in the lung study. The treatment portals were about the same, 20 cm by 20 cm; the dose a little bit higher, 2,000 to 2,500 rads in 10 days. We utilized a perineal portal as well to boost an additional 500 rads. There was absolutely no difference in the results between nonirradiated and the irradiated groups using the low dose scheme.

STEPHENS: Dr. PAULSON, will you tell us what happened to the five patients where the diagnosis was incorrect? Did the radiation therapy hasten their deaths, or did they survive?

PAULSON: Of the 5 patients, 3 had tuberculosis, 2 had metastatic adenocarcinomas. These 2 cases later developed evidence of a primary carcinoma in the colon. Whether the lesion in the lung was metastatic or an associated lesion we were not sure; we simply excluded them from the series. The 3 cases that were tuberculosis were recognized at the time of surgery, resected, continued on antimicrobial therapy with no deleterious effect from the radiation therapy they had received. With experience we have become more expert at diagnosing these, and if they are not absolutely typical as far as the pain is concerned, we cover them with antimicrobial therapy and then give them radiation therapy. Most patients with this carcinoma have characteristic severe pain with ulnar distribution. We feel that if we operate and find that it is carcinoma, we have jeopardized the patient's chance for cure. If we discover that it is tuberculosis, we would like to have had them on a medical management for a period of 4 to 6 weeks. We believe we are having our cake both ways in this instance. While there is a definite risk in this approach, we believe with experience we can make a clinical diagnosis with a high degree of accuracy.

STEPHENS: Most thoracic surgeons in the past have treated these patients with irradiation only. The irradiation retards the tumor, but the tumor regrows if not handled surgically as Dr. PAULSON recommends. Dr. ROSWIT, I think that you are dealing with 2 different types of people in spite of the fact that you have the same number that came to resection. Sixty of these patients died during the treatment period, which suggests to me that they were already disseminated. I know as a thoracic surgeon that diagnosis of carcinoma alone is not always easy. I just feel that in your operative group the cases were the kind that were asymptomatic and gave the best 5-year results anyhow.

ROSWIT: I would like to speak on the problem that Dr. Stephens has raised. These patients are about as comparable as two peas in a pod. We did everything possible in modern experimental design to guarantee this fact. There is a long delay; it takes 4 to 5 weeks to treat the patient, and then we have to wait 4 to 6 weeks before he can be operated on. So delay is a factor; but even more important is the dose given the patient. True, those who get a higher dose have a longer treatment period and there is a little more delay in such cases, but the dose seemed to be most important. In fact, I am grateful to my colleagues who gave the higher dose because now we have some facts that help us determine what ought to be the optimum dose. Dr. PAULSON, I think, was wise in selecting 3,000 rads in his series. I once made a worldwide questionnaire, asking for surviving bronchogenic carcinomas, 5 and 10 years, and nearly all of them had had dose levels of the order of 4,000 rads. Yes, these two groups (treated and control) are comparable. Some refused the operation, some developed metastases.

In the second study that I presented last year of the localized inoperable cases, we tested radiation therapy against the sugar tablet (lactose) and against chemicals. There are now over 1,000 patients in that study, which is still going on. We no longer are using lactose. Eighty-five to 92% are dead of distant metastases. The patient is at the mercy of his disease. We could end this cancer overnight, if we could give up our dearly beloved cigarettes. The fact is, we have to deal with the patients who are already here. Ninety-two percent of the metastatic cases were of the anaplastic oat cell type. The British reported in *Lancet* last month a 5-year study, testing radiation therapy versus surgery in such cases. In operable lung cancer, oat cell undifferentiated only, the irradiated cases came out better. So much better, in fact, that they are asking the surgeons of the British Empire not to operate on the oat cell tumor.

RUBIN: I was very curious, Dr. ROSWIT, in the figures that you presented to us; there is a no-difference kind of result to your overall series, the randomization data comparing the X-irradiated surgery group with the surgery group. The other manipulation of your data of moving one group to the point of resection, I think doesn't really give us any more information other than being disappointed with the outcome, so I think that was a valid kind of move. One would hope for some improvement. However, when you compare again the surgical group with the irradiated and resected group, you show clearly that there is a diminution in survival. This must mean that there is some group in the X-irradiated resected series that is doing better, in order to account for the fact that the two were similar at the beginning. The only group that you haven't perhaps identified clearly is the group that was just irradiated, and for some reason never came for surgery. That means that that group must have done very well in order to bring the figure back up to the control value which might substantiate in some degree some of the British studies. In other words, in the operable patients, it could well be that whether you used surgery or irradiation, the outcome may indeed be very similar. The problem here may be that the combination of two forms of therapy is more detrimental than either one alone.

Roswit: The 1-year figures for those that had irradiation, but no operation have the same survival as those patients who had nothing done. The controls were people who never came to surgery; and giving radiation therapy or doing nothing is about the same for that group, believe it or not.

Rubin: Nevertheless, Dr. Roswit, in order to explain the difference between these two groups, there must be one group in the X-irradiated and surgerized series that is bringing these values back to the baseline. I'm trying to identify this and I can't from the data you have presented. Clearly there's something here which is lacking.

Roswit: In our localized inoperable study, all histologically identical, which runs about 1,000 patients now, we compared radiation therapy with Cytoxan chemotherapy; at one year 25% of the irradiated are surviving. They are given 4,000 to 5,000 rads of high energy radiations. Only 15% of the Cytoxan cases survive, which is no better than doing nothing at all. We're dropping that drug, except for one kind of cancer, the oat cell or anaplastic tumor. There's a very significant improvement in survival, in both the disseminated and localized inoperable, for this particular drug, the only drug of all the dozens we've tried.

Front. Radiation Ther. Onc., vol. 5, pp. 188–197
(Karger, Basel/München/Paris/New York 1970)

Preoperative Radiation Therapy
in the Management of Breast Cancer[1]

G. H. FLETCHER, E. D. MONTAGUE, and E. C. WHITE

Department of Radiotherapy, The University of Texas, M. D. Anderson Hospital and
Tumor Institute at Houston, Houston, Tex.

The management of breast cancer, whether by surgical procedures or irradiation, has two purposes, with the emphasis somewhat varying according to the stage of disease; first, absolute cure by eradication either surgically or radiotherapeutically of every cancer cell, thereby preventing appearance of disease at any time after the original treatment; second, local control of the primary tumor and of the spread to the regional lymphatics.

The 10-year survival rate is an important basis for assessing success when dealing with breast cancer patients because at 10 years the cumulative death rate becomes parallel to the one for patients without cancer. This is in contradistinction to squamous cell carcinoma, where a 5-year survival is a reliable indication of permanent cure.

The role of radiation therapy in the primary treatment of patients with breast cancer is to be evaluated from the standpoint of survival rates and incidence of recurrences within the irradiated area.

This essay is limited to the analysis of the indications, techniques, and results in patients who receive preoperative irradiation prior to radical mastectomy.

[1] This investigation was supported by Public Health Service Research Grants No. CA-06294 and CA-05654 from the National Cancer Institute.

Treatment Categories

A protocol sheet with diagrams is completed for each patient with breast cancer at The University of Texas M. D. Anderson Hospital and Tumor Institute at Houston. Using this description of the clinical features of the disease, one can retrospectively fit the cases into any staging system, except those cases where an open biopsy was performed elsewhere and there is subsequent hematoma and/or infection and staging is impossible. Table I shows the clinical criteria which have evolved at our institution from 1948 to 1964 to determine the modalities of definitivetreatment [3].

Those patients referred with disturbed biopsy sites (hematomas, ecchymosis, infection) or with clinical features listed in Category II are treated with Cobalt-60 preoperative irradiation followed by radical mastectomy 5 to 6 weeks later.

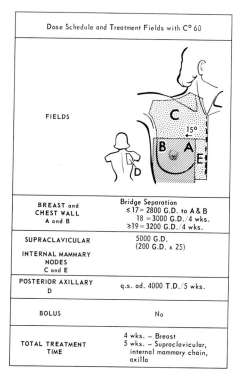

Dose Schedule and Treatment Fields with C° 60	
FIELDS	
BREAST and CHEST WALL A and B	Bridge Separation ≤17= 2800 G.D. to A & B 18 = 3000 G.D./4 wks. ≥19 = 3200 G.D./4 wks.
SUPRACLAVICULAR INTERNAL MAMMARY NODES C and E	5000 G.D. (200 G.D. x 25)
POSTERIOR AXILLARY D	q.s. ad. 4000 T.D./5 wks.
BOLUS	No
TOTAL TREATMENT TIME	4 wks. – Breast 5 wks. – Supraclavicular, internal mammary chain, axilla

Fig. 1. Schematic drawings of portals and treatment schedules.

Table I. Categories[1] of treatment for breast cancer

	I	II	III	IV
	Radical mastectomy outer quadrant and axilla (—): no post-operative irradiation. Others: periph. lymph. irradiation	Preoperative irradiation + radical mastectomy[2]	Clinically unsuitable for rad. mastectomy. Radical irradiation or simple mastectomy+radical irradiation	Technically unsuitable for radical mastectomy. Occasionally radical irradiation, usually rapid palliative irradiation
Primary Size	<5 cm	>5 cm	<Whole breast	Whole breast
Skin	—	Edema or fixation over tumor only	Edema, ulceration, skin fixation <½ breast. Satellite nodules in continuity with primary. Inflammatory with limited { erythema, peau d'orange, ridges	Edema, ulceration, skin fixation } >½ breast. Peripheral satellite nodules. Massive inflammatory
Pect. fascia+chest wall	—	—	Pectoral fascia fixation	Chest wall fixation
Axillary nodes Size	<2 cm	>2 cm or few	Large, with or without limited fixation or multiple or apical	Massive, fixed
Number	Single			
Location	Not apical	Not apical		

Supraclavicular nodes	—	—	Moveable	Fixed
Staging UICC	T_1 (N_0, N_1) T_2 (N_0, N_1)	T_1, N_1 $(+)$ T_2 $(+)$ (N_0, N_1)	T_3 (N_0, N_1) (T_1, T_2) N_2 (T_1, T_2) N_3 (infra- or supraclavicular)	(T_1, T_2, T_3) N_3 T_4 (N_0, N_1, N_2, N_3)
American Joint Committee	(T_1, T_2) (N_0, N_1)	T_2 $(+)$ $(N_0, N_1$ $(+))$	T_3 (N_0, N_1) (T_1, T_2) N_2 M (supraclavicular)	T_3 $(+)$ (N_0, N_1, N_2) (T_1, T_2) $(N_2$ $(+))$ M (supraclavicular)

T_x $(+)$, or N_x $(+)$: late x.
T_x (N_y, N_z): T_xN_y and T_xN_z.

[1] The worst feature places the patient in the appropriate category. Multiple features in one category do not change the category.
[2] Also patients with outside open biopsy and a disturbed wound.

Courtesy: Fletcher et al. [5].

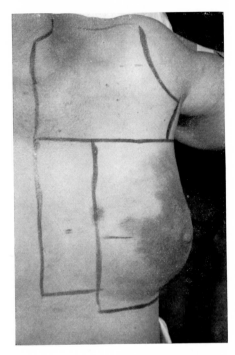

Fig. 2. Portals drawn on a patient with a separate internal mammary chain field. The area of ecchymosis is covered entirely.

Technique of Preoperative Irradiation

Since 1954 Cobalt-60 has been used exclusively. The irradiated area covers the chest wall, the axilla, supraclavicular area, and internal mammary chain. Figure 1 shows the schematic drawings of the portals; figure 2 shows the fields drawn on a patient with extensive ecchymosis; figure 3 shows the patient in treatment position on the Cobalt-60 teletherapy unit.

A radical mastectomy is performed 6 weeks following completion of irradiation with no apparent increased difficulty on the part of the surgeon. In fact, the interstitial edema which is present often makes easier the surgical dissection. There is no increase in wound healing complications (table II).

Supraclavicular area and axilla. The anterior supraclavicular-axillary portal (C) received 5,000 rads given dose in 25 treatments of 200 rads each. The posterior portal is given q.s. for 4,000 rads at midaxilla in five weeks.

Corpus mammae. No bolus is used to ensure maximum skin sparing.

A given dose of 2,800 rads is delivered to each tangential field for a bridge separation of 17 cm or less, 3,000 rads given dose for 18 cm. In those patients in whom additional span of breast bridge is necessary in order to avoid splitting an inner quadrant lesion, a breast span greater than 18 cm will be necessary. Then 3,200 rads are given to each of the tangential fields.

Internal mammary chain. Ordinarily, if a bridge separation is greater than 18 cm, a separate internal mammary field is used.

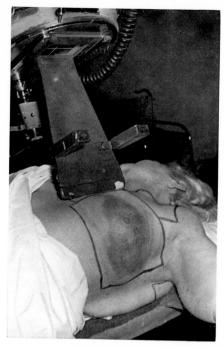

Fig. 3. Patient in treatment position. Medial tangential field placement.

Table II. Relationship between wound healing following radical mastectomy and 5 days
a week treatment

	Preoperative irradiation Cobalt-60	Radical mastectomy first
Number of patients	211	534
Delayed wound healing	3	18
Moderate slough	23	43
Severe slough with skin graft	3	11
Rib necrosis	1	1
Wound infection	1	0

Modified from. FLETCHER *et al.* [2].

A tumor dose of 4,500 rads is delivered at a 3 cm depth at a rate of 1,000 rads TD per week or possibly up to 5,000 rads in medial tumors and palpable axillary nodes and/or with primaries greater than 5 cm.

In those patients without a separate internal mammary field, a supplementary internal mammary field is used on completion of treatment of the tangential fields to raise the tumor dose to the entire internal mammary chain to 4,500 rads.

Results

Table III gives the survival rates at 5 and 10 years. The highest 10-year survival rate is in the preoperative group.

Table IV gives the 5- and 10-year survival rates by the two subcategories (borderline operable and disturbed breast and axillary nodes palpable and nonpalpable). The survival rates at 5 and 10 years, primarily at 10 years for the borderline operable group are suggestive of the effectiveness of preoperative irradiation.

Table III. Survival and NED rates in patients having had a radical mastectomy (Jan. 1948– Dec. 1964)

Modality	No. of patients	5- year survival per cent [1]	10-year survival per cent [1]
Radical Mastectomy [2]	982	64.0 [3]	50.0 [4]
Alone	283	70.0	55.5
With postop. irradiation	364	56.0	38.0
With preop. irradiation	335	68.5	60.5

[1] Berkson-Gage.
[2] 25% private; 42% clinic; 33% indigent.
[3] Outer quadrants 62.0%; inner quadrants and central 66.5%.
[4] Outer quadrants 50.5%; inner quadrants and central 50.5%.

Table IV. Preoperative irradiation percentage 5-and 10-year survival rates [1] (Jan. 1948– Dec. 1965)

	No. of patients	Palpable ax. nodes		Nonpalpable ax. nodes	
		5 years	10 years	5 years	10 years
Borderline operable	66	51	43	70	56
Open biopsy (281) Probable tumorectomy (38)	319	66.5	58	73.5	67

[1] Berkson-Gage.

Table V shows the incidence of recurrences. The low incidence in the disturbed breast group shows that irradiation does not produce recurrences, contrary to another report [1]. A 12-per cent incidence in the borderline operability group is low considering the advanced stage of the lesions [6].

Table V. Preoperative irradiation of carcinoma of breast sites of recurrence (Jan. 1948–Dec. 1965)

Site of recurrence[1]	Borderline operable (66) axillary nodes on admission		Biopsied (281) or tumorectomies (38) axillary nodes on admission	
	Palpable (49)	Nonpalpable (17)	Palpable (171)	Nonpalpable (148)
Chest wall	6 (12%)	2 (12%)	5%	1.5%
Axilla	0	0	0.6%	0%
Supraclavicular	2	1	2%	1.5%
Parasternal	1	0	0%	0.7%

[1] Multiple sites of recurrences are counted for each site.

Table VI. Control rates of nonpalpable axillary and supraclavicular disease

Incidence of recurrence			
Axilla (Jan. 1959–Dec. 1964)	Supraclavicular area (Jan. 1948–Dec. 1964)		
Category III patients 52 5,000 rads TD in 5 weeks with Cobalt-60	Axilla+in specimen of radical mastectomy no Postop Irrad. Manchester[2] Memorial NYC[2]	Axilla+in specimen of radical mastectomy and pre- or postop irrad. MDAH 699 patients	Category III & IV patients 491 without palpable supraclav. nodes on admission 5,000 rads skin dose/ 12 weeks with 250 Kv 5,000 rads given dose/5 weeks with Cobalt-60
NED Disease CW[1] CW[1]			
46 6 Failure 0 2	20–25%	≤3,500 rads, 250 Kv in 3–4 weeks 7% 4,000–4,500 rads Co-60 in 4 weeks 2%	3.5%

[1] CW = Chest Wall.
[2] Jackson [7], Robbins *et al.* [8].

Discussion

From the incidence of supraclavicular disease in our material and the incidence in the Manchester and Memorial Hospital series (tables V-VI), one can conclude that doses of 3,000 to 3,500 rads in 3 weeks can control approximately 70% of subclinical aggregates of cancer cells and 4,000 to 4,500 rads in 4 weeks or 5,000 rads in 5 weeks can control 90% of them [4]. There were 95 of 366 Category III patients who had no palpable axillary nodes. Because of the advanced disease in the breast one would expect at least 30% of these patients to have axillary node involvement. With a TD of 5,000 rads in 5 weeks, only two patients, who also had a failure at the primary site, developed axillary disease. These data show the great differences in doses necessary to sterilize subclinical breast cancer because 9,000 to 10,000 rads may fail to sterilize large masses. The objection levelled to pre- or postoperative irradiation that doses of the order of 4,000 to 5,000 rads in 4 to 5 weeks could not be effective has been removed.

Although the clinical material was not randomized and, therefore, the conclusions are not absolute, preoperative irradiation appears to produce a diminution in the incidence of local recurrences and possibly improves survival rates. When proper megavoltage techniques are used, the problems of wound healing are the same as when primary radical mastectomy is performed first.

Since 1965, there is a trend to prefer simple mastectomy with dissection of palpable nodes in the borderline operable cases, as there is indication that survival and local control rates are equally as good with the more conservative surgical procedure.

References

1. DAO, T. L. and KOVARIC, J. P.: Incidence of pulmonary and skin metastases in women with breast cancer who received postoperative irradiation. Surgery 52: 203–212 (1962).
2. FLETCHER, G. H.; WHITE, E. C., and MONTAGUE, E. D.: Evaluation of preoperative irradiation for carcinoma of the breast; in Proceedings Fifth National Cancer Conference, pp. 469–474 (Lippincott, Philadelphia 1965).
3. FLETCHER, G. H.: Primary management of breast cancer; in Textbook of Radiotherapy, pp. 336–359 (Lea & Febiger, Philadelphia 1966).
4. FLETCHER, G. H.; MONTAGUE, E. D., and WHITE, E. C.: Evaluation of irradiation of the peripheral lymphatics in conjunction with radical mastectomy for breast cancer. Cancer 21 : 791–797 (1968).

5. FLETCHER, G. H.; MONTAGUE, E. D., and WHITE, E. C.: Role of radiation therapy in the primary management of breast cancer; in ARIEL Progress in clinical cancer, pp. 242–256 (Grune & Stratton, New York, 1969).
6. SPRATT, J. S.: Locally recurrent cancer after radical mastectomy. Cancer 20: 1,051–1,053 (1967).
7. JACKSON, S. M.: Carcinoma of the breast – The significance of supraclavicular lymph node metastases. Clin. Radiol. 17: 107 (1966).
8. ROBBINS, G. F.; LUCAS, J. C.; FRACCHIA, A. A.; FARROW, J. H., and CHU, F. G. H.: An evaluation of postoperative prophylactic radiation therapy in breast cancer. Surg. Gynec. Obstet. 122: 979 (1966).

Authors' addresses: Dr. GILBERT H. FLETCHER, Head, Department of Radiotherapy, The University of Texas, M. D. Anderson Hospital and Tumor Institute, Houston, TX 77025; Dr. ELEANOR D. MONTAGUE, Radiotherapist, Department of Radiotherapy, Methodist Hospital, 6516 Bertner, Houston, TX 77025; Dr. EDGAR C. WHITE, Head, Department of Surgery, The University of Texas, M. D. Anderson Hospital and Tumor Institute, Houston, TX 77025 (USA).

Front. Radiation Ther. Onc., vol. 5, pp. 198–205
(Karger, Basel/München/Paris/New York 1970)

Simple Mastectomy and Radical Radiation Therapy in Cancer of the Breast

R. McWHIRTER

In the past thirty years there has been a dramatic change in our whole outlook in the management of breast cancer. Thirty years ago the classical Halsted operation was the undisputed method of treatment. So firmly was this belief held, that when it was first suggested there might be other methods worthy of consideration, the suggestion was regarded almost as an act of heresy. Nevertheless other methods were introduced and these are now so numerous and so diverse that we have great difficulty in deciding which method of treatment is best. This remarkable change of outlook might be expressed somewhat differently by saying that we have departed from a haven of security and having passed through the turbulent waters at the harbour bar we now find ourselves adrift in a sea of uncertainty.

This state of uncertainty arose because the basis on which different methods of treatment were compared was often unsatisfactory. The error most commonly made, was comparison by survival rates without regard to the extent of the disease treated. This led to much confusion and, as the error still continues to be made, it is worth emphasising at this point that the extent of disease treated may have a much greater influence on the survival rates than the method of treatment employed. Clinical trials, to which reference will be made later, have now become the accepted method of evaluating different forms of treatment.

Radical Mastectomy

Radical mastectomy is the obvious starting point in any discussion. Introduced at the turn of the century, radical mastectomy is still the method in most common use.

Many more patients now seek advice at an earlier stage of the disease and accordingly a higher proportion can now be treated by radical mastectomy. Now if a method of treatment is effective and is employed in a higher proportion of patients we would expect to find a fall in the mortality rates. Our national statistics however show that the mortality rate from breast cancer is the same today as it was at the beginning of the century. It is not surprising therefore that the value of radical mastectomy has been called in question.

It is true that the survival rates from radical mastectomy are now much higher but this is not necessarily an indication that progress has been made. The higher survival rates could be due entirely to the fact that patients with advanced disease are no longer treated by radical mastectomy. There is good evidence that patients are now being more carefully selected for the operation. Thus we find, in centres where statistics have been kept over a long period of time, that the proportion of patients with positive nodes has fallen from around 60% to about 40% or even lower.

The results when the axillary nodes are negative have always been good but negative nodes are not a test of the value of axillary dissection. The real test comes when the nodes are positive and the results are then always much lower. The high failure rate when axillary dissection is really required is one of the main reasons for suggesting that other methods should be considered.

The More Radical Approach

HANDLEY's findings [5] in respect of the internal mammary nodes are well known. His observations have been confirmed by many surgeons and the internal mammary nodes are now accepted as being part of the regional lymph node drainage system of the breast. It has been shown that by the time the axillary nodes are invaded, the internal mammary nodes are also invaded in about 50% of patients. In addition it has been demonstrated by biopsy of the supraclavicular nodes and by follow up studies after radical mastectomy that the supraclavicular nodes are also commonly involved by the time the axillary nodes are invaded. Both obser-

vations help to explain why the survival rates are low in patients
with positive axillary nodes.

When the internal mammary and supraclavicular nodes are
invaded, standard radical mastectomy does not offer any chance
of cure. Recognising this point, Haagensen [4] now carries
out a biopsy of the internal mammary nodes and of the apical
axillary nodes before accepting a patient for treatment by radical
mastectomy. We must note however, that restriction of the field
of treatment will not cure more patients. The alternative approach
is to extend the field of treatment to include the internal mammary
and supraclavicular nodes. This approach may not be successful
but it must be attempted if we are to try to reduce the mortality
rate in breast cancer.

The feasibility of complete surgical excision of the internal
mammary and supraclavicular nodes was examined by Wangensteen [11] but the high morbidity and mortality associated with
this extensive operation suggest that it is unlikely to become the
routine method of treating breast cancer.

In an operation associated with little or no morbidity, Urban
[10] has resected the internal mammary nodes in continuity with
the breast. The results he has obtained encourage the belief that
distant metastases are not always present when the internal mammary nodes are involved and that extension of treatment beyond
the scope of the standard radical operation is worth undertaking.

Supplementation of the standard radical operation by radiotherapy directed to the internal mammary and supraclavicular
nodes has been widely undertaken. The value of radiotherapy,
given immediately ofter radical mastectomy, was examined by
Paterson and Russell [9] who found that the survival rates
were no better than those obtained when radiotherapy was given
only if and when local recurrence took place. In Edinburgh from
1935–40, radiotherapy was given routinely immediately after radical mastectomy. The local recurrence rate was markedly reduced
but infortunately there was little improvement in the five year
survival rate.

In 1941, following a discussion with the senior surgical staff
of Edinburgh Royal Infirmary, it was decided to substitute radiotherapy for surgery in the treatment of the regional lymph nodes.
A clinical trial was proposed but was rejected because in those

days any trial involving patients was not considered to be ethical. At a time when radical mastectomy was the unchallenged method of treatment it was admittedly a bold decision to substitute radio- therapy for surgery in the treatment of the lymph nodes and some account must be given for the reasons leading up to this decision. KEYNES [7] had shown earlier that radium implantation of the regional nodes yielded results comparable to surgical dissection and it was thought that X-ray treatment might be even more effective because of the much better dose distribution. X-ray treat- ment had already been shown to be effective in the treatment of local recurrence. Immediate radiotherapy after radical mastectomy had markedly reduced the incidence of local recurrences on the chest wall and parasternal masses due to internal mammary node involvement became exceedingly uncommon. In a small number of patients treated by simple mastectomy and radiotherapy in the period 1935–40 the results were encouraging. The decision had the full support of the late Sir JOHN FRASER [2] who had recently reviewed the patients he had treated by radical mastec- tomy and had found that the survival rates, especially in patients with positive nodes, were disappointing. We were also encouraged by the fact that the new method of treatment would offer exactly the same prospect of cure as radical mastectomy if the axillary nodes were negative (excision of negative axillary nodes cannot modify the survival rate). The decision to continue to remove the breast before irradiating the nodes was based on the findings in patients with advanced disease who had been treated entirely by radiotherapy. In these patients the response in the nodes was always much better than in the breast and, indeed, it was only rarely that the primary tumour disappeared entirely.

With few exceptions (axillary tail tumours, lymph nodes in continuity with the primary tumour, patients with pulmonary tuberculosis and patients with peripheral vascular disease of the arm) simple mastectomy and radiotherapy could be undertaken in all patients suitable for the standard radical operation. It was soon found that full treatment by this means could also be given to patients with fixed axillary nodes and palpable supraclavicular nodes – a group of patients in whom radical treatment had hith- erto been impossible. Treatment by this means accordingly offered a chance of cure to many more patients.

The crude survival rates are presented in table I. The patients
have been classified according to the International form of staging
adopted in 1960 and the analysis has been confined to patients
under 65 years of age so as to minimise the effect of death from
intercurrent disease in the long term survival rates.

Table I. All patients under 65 years treated by simple mastectomy and radical radiotherapy
(deaths from intercurrent disease included)

		No. of cases	Percentage alive		
			5 years	10 years	15 years
Stage I	T.1 N.0	206	79	64	47
	T.2 N.0	394	68	48	40
	Total	600	72	54	43
Stage II	T.1 N.1	116	67	51	43
	T.2 N.1	375	55	41	32
	Total	491	58	43	35
Stage III	Total	690	37	24	17

Review of Methods Discussed

Reviewing all the methods of treatment which have been discussed,
we find the position is less complex than it might appear at first sight.

It will be noted that, so far as the primary tumour is concerned,
there appears to be general agreement that surgical removal of
the breast is the best form of treatment.

When we come to the treatment of the lymph nodes, however,
we find a difference of opinion but in view of the agreement on
the treatment of the disease in the breast an interesting observation can be made. In patients in whom all the regional lymph
nodes are negative the survival rates will be the same for all the
various methods of treatment which have been discussed (whether
negative nodes are treated by surgery or radiotherapy is of no
importance, the survival rates will be unaffected by either form
of treatment).

Unfortunately clinical assessment of the state of the nodes is
inaccurate and accordingly we must treat all nodes to ensure that
positive nodes will not escape treatment.

We must first try to decide whether treatment should be limited to the axillary nodes, as in the standard radical operation, or extended to include the internal mammary and supraclavicular nodes as well. We can assume that as the extent of lymph node involvement increases, the frequency of distant metastases will also increase. If distant metastases are present in all patients with internal mammary and/or supraclavicular involvement then there is no indication for extended treatment. But we do not know if this is so and I have shown previously, even when the supraclavicular nodes are palpable and therefore grossly involved, that a five year survival rate of 17% can be obtained when these nodes are radically treated by radiotherapy [8]. In a series of 123 patients who were clinically operable but who had been found to have metastatic disease in the lymph nodes at the apex of the axilla or in the internal mammary nodes, GUTTMANN [3], employing two million volt radiotherapy as the sole means of treatment, obtained a five year survival rate of 52%. Extension of treatment to include the internal mammary and supraclavicular nodes would therefore appear to be worthy of further consideration.

The remaining point which must be resolved is the actual method of treatment of the lymph nodes. Should the nodes be treated by surgery or by radiotherapy? Treatment of one group of nodes (the axillary group) by surgery and the other nodes (the internal mammary and supraclavicular) by radiotherapy does not assist in the solution of the problem. The position will remain confused until we can decide on one or other method of treatment for all lymph nodes.

There are, of course, other problems but it would appear from the discussion that the two main problems requiring solution are as follows: (1) Should the lymph nodes be treated by surgery or radiotherapy? (2) should all the regional lymph nodes be treated (as in the extended methods) or only the axillary group (as in the standard radical operation)?

Clinical Trials

Clinical trials are now the accepted method of resolving a difference of opinion. Some trials have already been completed.

In a trial undertaken by KAAE and JOHANSEN [6], extended radical mastectomy was compared with simple mastectomy and radiotherapy. No significant difference was found in the survival rates or in the recurrence-free rates.

In a trial confined to patients with Stage II carcinomas, BRINKLEY and HAYBITTLE [1] compared standard radical mastectomy and radiotherapy with simple mastectomy and radiotherapy and found a marginal difference in favour of the latter method.

As already stated, PATERSON and RUSSELL [9] undertook a trial in patients previously treated by standard radical mastectomy and compared radiotherapy given shortly after the operation with radiotherapy delivered only when recurrences developed. They reported no significant difference in the survival rates but noted that routine post-operative radiotherapy markedly inhibited the incidence of local recurrence.

So far these trials and others undertaken to determine the best method of hormone management, have shown little or no difference in the value of the methods compared. To some extent this is what might have been anticipated because trials are undertaken only where doubt exists and are never undertaken when one method is obviously better than another. From what has been said earlier, it is highly probable that any difference in the value of two methods of treatment will be confined to one or more sub-groups of the patients treated and this difference may be difficult to detect unless refined methods of analysis are employed and the numbers in the sub-groups are adequate to permit of a valid comparison. Clinical trials are certainly not a simple means of solving our difficulties but our experience in their design and interpretation is steadily improving and there can be little doubt that we can look forward to a time when the treatment of breast cancer will no longer be in a state of uncertainty.

Summary

The many different methods of treatment introduced in recent years have created great uncertainty regarding the treatment of breast cancer. Two major problems require solution. We must decide whether treatment should be extended to include the internal mammary and supraclavicular nodes. We must also decide between surgery and radiotherapy in the treatment of the lymph nodes. Well designed clinical trials afford the best means of resolving these problems.

References

1. BRINKLEY, D. and HAYBITTLE, J. L.: Treatment of stage II carcinoma of the female breast. Lancet 2: 291–295 (1966).
2. FRASER, J.: Some reflections on pathogenesis and treatment of cancer of breast (Honyman Gillespie Lecture) Edinburgh med. J. 46: 509–528 (1939).
3. GUTTMANN, R. J.: Role of supervoltage irradiation of regional lymph node bearing areas in breast cancer. Amer. J. Roentgenol. 96: 560–564 (1966).
4. HAAGENSEN, C. E.: Diseases of the breast (Saunders, Philadelphia 1956).
5. HANDLEY, R. S. and THACKRAY, A. C.: Invasion of the internal mammary lymph glands in carcinoma of the breast. Brit. J. Cancer 1: 15–20 (1947).
6. KAAE, S. and JOHANSEN, H.: Simple versus radical mastectomy in primary breast cancer. Prognostic factors in breast cancer. Proceedings of first tenovus symposium, pp. 93–102 (Livingstone, Edinburgh 1967).
7. KEYNES, G.: Conservative treatment of cancer of the breast. Brit. med. J. 2: 643–653 (1937).
8. McWHIRTER, R.: Should more radical treatment be attempted in breast cancer? Amer. J. Roentgenol. 92: 3–13 (1964).
9. PATERSON, R. and RUSSELL, M. H.: Clinical trials in malignant disease-III-breast cancer. J. Fac. Radiol. 10: 175–180 (1959).
10. URBAN, J. A.: Clinical experience and results of excision of internal mammary lymph node chain in primary operable breast cancer. Cancer. 12: 14–22 (1959).
11. WANGENSTEEN, O. H.: Proceedings of the Second International Cancer Conference, Cincinnati, vol. 1, pp. 230–239 (1952).

Author's address: Prof. Robert McWHIRTER, Department of Radiotherapy, Royal Infirmary, Edinburgh, EH3 9YW (Scotland).

Front. Radiation Ther. Onc., vol. 5, pp. 206–230
(Karger, Basel/München/Paris/New York 1970)

Postoperative Radiotherapy
in the Treatment of Breast Cancer

T. L. DAO and T. W. HSIA

Department of Breast Surgery, Roswell Park Memorial Institute, New York State Department
of Health, Buffalo, N. Y.

I. Introduction

For some years now, the value of postoperative radiotherapy in the treatment of breast cancer has been a subject of controversy. Proponents of postoperative radiotherapy believe that irradiation can 'destroy' or 'sterilize' the field containing mammary cancer cells that are 'disseminated' during surgery or 'left behind' by incomplete dissection. Opponents reason conceptually that carcinoma of the breast is a systemic disease which cannot be cured by local treatment. They further insist that cancer cells cannot be entirely destroyed by irradiation.

Several well-designed and carefully-controlled studies have been carried out to determine the value of ionizing irradiation after radical mastectomy in the treatment of carcinoma of the breast. PATERSON and RUSSELL [7] reported that there were no differences in mortality rate at 5 years in two groups of patients (a total of 1,461); 709 patients had postoperative irradiation and the other group of 752, radical mastectomy alone. EASSON [4] presented a critical analysis of the original series of 1,461 patients followed up for a minimum period of ten years after their treatment. The conclusion was that X-ray therapy following Halsted radical mastectomy did not prevent death from metastases, and that there was advantage to the patient in avoiding prophylactic radiation therapy.

A prospective randomized clinical trial to evaluate the therapeutic value of postoperative radiotherapy in the treatment of breast cancer has also been undertaken by the National Surgical Adjuvant Chemotherapy Breast Cancer Study Group. The preliminary analysis of the study shows that there is no difference in either the mortality or the recurrence rate between the two groups of patients, one receiving ionizing radiation shortly after the radical mastectomy and the other, radical mastectomy alone. The complete results of this study will be published soon.

In spite of the well-designed and executed Manchester study [7], the consensus among the American radiotherapists and surgeons is that postoperative radiotherapy in patients with regional nodal metastases may reduce the incidence of 'local' recurrence and perhaps delay onset of distant metastases. In the present study, we wish to determine whether postoperative radiotherapy in stage II breast cancer can (1) reduce the incidence of 'local' recurrence, (2) delay the appearance of metastases, thus prolonging the 'metastases-free' interval, and, (3) influence the pattern of subsequent metastases.

II. ˙Mechanism of the Study

A. Criteria for Inclusion of Cases in this Study
The cases included in this study must meet the following criteria.

1. They all must have had a radical mastectomy (Halsted procedure) for an operable breast cancer.

2. The axillary lymph nodes removed at the time of radical mastectomy must be proved to contain metastases by microscopic examination.

3. There must have been no clinical evidence of presence of supraclavicular metastases at the time of mastectomy.

4. Radiotherapy must be given within 3 to 4 weeks of radical mastectomy.

5. The field of irradiation must include the supraclavicular, the axilla and the parasternal regions. The radiation dosage must be 2,500 R or above for any portal if a conventional high voltage machine is used.

6. There must be no other concomitant therapy at the time of mastectomy and radiotherapy.

7. All of the patients must have had either primary or secondary adrenalectomy for treatment of their metastases.

B. An Analysis of the Technique of Radiotherapy Used in the Study Cases
Conventional high voltage radiotherapy was used in the majority of the patients; only 6 of 86 patients received Cobalt 60 therapy. The radiation technique used in these patients is remarkably uniform, both in dosage and fields of irradiation. It can be summarized as follows:

Quality: 200, 220, and 250 KVP machines were used with HVL 0.5 to 2.0 mm Cu for most patients.

Fields: The fields included in the postoperative radiotherapy were uniform; they were (1) direct anterior chest wall (internal mammary area), and (2) anterior and posterior supra-clavicular fields including the apex of the axilla.

Dosage: For anterior chest wall (internal mammary region) the total dosage used in this series of patients ranged from 2,500 to 3,600 R; for the anterior and posterior supraclavicular including the axillary ports, the dosage ranged from 3,000 to 4,000 R to each port. In the majority of cases, the total radiation dosage for each of the supraclavicular and axillary portal was 3,500 R.

Duration of radiation program: Irradiation was delivered over a period of 3 to 4 weeks.

Cobalt 60 gamma radiation was used in only 6 of the 86 patients. The technique was essentially similar. The areas of irradiation included the parasternal area for internal mammary nodes and the axilla and the supraclavicular fossa in continuity. The radiation dosages were higher than those given with the conventional high voltage machine. They ranged from 3,750 to 6,400 R per field.

III. Results of the Study

A. Clinical Materials

This study is based on a retrospective analysis of a series of 262 consecutive cases of breast cancer referred to the breast service at Roswell Park Memorial Institute between January 1962 and December 1967 inclusive, for treatment of metastases when first discovered. Of this entire series, 118 patients had ionizing radiations after radical mastectomy and 144 had radical mastectomy only. Critical analysis of the results was made for 176 patients; 86 had radical mastectomy and postoperative radiotherapy and 90 had radical mastectomy only. The remaining 86 were excluded for one of the following reasons: (1) axillary nodes were negative in 72 patients, (2) 9 patients received concomitant therapy such as surgical or radiation castration, (3) 'inadequate radiation dosage' was used in 2 patients, and (4) 3 patients had incomplete follow-ups. The two groups of patients were comparable in both their age ranges and their menstrual status. The age of the patients in the group receiving radical mastectomy alone ranged from 35 to 73, with a median of 53 and a mean of 53.4. There were 26 pre-menopausal and 64 post-menopausal patients in this group. The age of the patients in the radical mastectomy and postoperative radiotherapy group ranged from 34 to 73 with a median of 55 and a mean of 53.5. There were 23 premenopausal and 67 post-menopausal patients in this group.

B. Incidence and Characteristics of Skin Metastases

Throughout this paper, the term 'skin metastasis' or 'skin recurrence', rather than 'local recurrence', is used to describe the

Table I. Incidence of skin metastases in patients with cancer of the breast

Type of treatment	Total No. of cases	Incidence of skin metastases		
		Initial occurrence	Late appearance	Total
Radical mastectomy only	90	39	6	45 (50%)
Radical mastectomy and postoperative radiotherapy	86	31	2	33 (37%)

Table II. Incidence of metastases to skin and other sites in patients with disseminated cancer of the breast

Type of Treatment	Total No. of cases	No. with skin metastases[1]	Chest wall only	Concomitant with other sites		
				Lungs	Bones	Others
Radical mastectomy only	90	39 (43%)	15	10	11	3
Radical mastectomy and postoperative radiotherapy	86	31 (35%)	13	14	4	–

[1] Only those having skin metastases as initial sign of recurrence.

appearance of skin lesions in the chest wall. The term 'local recurrence' is not descriptive of the pathological nature of skin lesions in the chest wall.

The data in table I demonstrate that the incidence of skin metastases in the chest wall is slightly lower in patients receiving postoperative radiotherapy: 39 out of 90 patients treated with radical mastectomy alone, and 31 out of 86 in those receiving radiation after mastectomy. The difference, however, is not statistically significant. The data in table II further show that more than half of the patients with skin metastases at the onset also have metastatic lesions elsewhere. It should be noted that the incidence of lung metastases in concomitance with skin metastases is higher in patients receiving postoperative irradiation than in those treated with mastectomy alone.

An interesting observation in this study is the remarkable difference in the pattern of skin metastases in the two groups of patients. We observed extensive dermal metastases, often limited to the areas of the superficial skin that had been exposed to radiation (fig. 1, 2). Whereas extensive anterior chest wall skin metastases were seen in only 2 of the 39 non-irradiated patients with skin recurrence, 11 of the 31 patients receiving postoperative irradiation showed this unusual phenomenon. In the overwhelming majority of non-irradiated patients, metastases were in the form of a few to multiple nodules scattered throughout the chest wall or along the operative scar. Cutaneous metastases in the posterior scapular region were never seen in non-irradiated patients but were observed in 8 of the 31 patients with skin metastases (fig. 3).

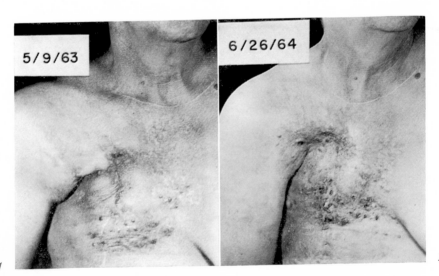

Fig. 1. Dermal metastases in the irradiated area in patient M. S. 14 months after radical mastectomy and postoperative radiotherapy.

Fig. 2. Progression of the metastases in the skin still confined to the area of X-irradiation. Note: Skin lesions are extending beyond the posterior axillary line to the back.

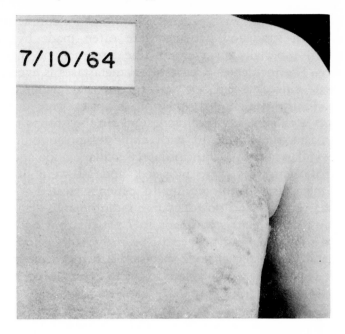

Fig. 3. Dermal metastases in the same patient extending up to the posterior scapular area and the neck.

When metastatic skin lesions in the chest wall appeared as the only evidence of recurrence of the disease, they were treated either with surgical excision or irradiation. Surgical excisions were done when skin lesions were few and limited to a small area that could be excised. Multiple skin lesions scattered over a larger area were treated with irradiation. Results in table III show that all 15 patients in the radical mastectomy group were treated, but only 9 of 13 patients in the mastectomy and postoperative radiotherapy group could be treated with either surgical excision or local irradiation. The remaining 4 patients had such extensive skin involvement that local treatment would be futile. It was further observed that the response rate to local therapy was considerably higher in skin metastases occurring in patients who did not receive postoperative radiotherapy.

Recurrence in regional lymph nodes is difficult to assess and any attempt to make quantitative analysis is unreliable. It is often difficult to palpate recurrent supraclavicular nodes in the extremely

Table V. Incidence of pulmonary metastases in irradiated and non-irradiated patients with breast cancer

Type of treatment	Total No. cases	No. of patients with pulmonary metastases[1]			
		Ipsilateral	Contralateral	Bilateral	Total
Radical mastectomy only	90	10	5	27	42 (46%)
Radical mastectomy and postoperative radiotherapy	86	18	5	27	50 (57%)

[1] Pulmonary metastases in patients who were dying of breast cancer.

D. *A Comparison of the 'Metastases-Free' Interval and the Survival Rate*

An analysis of the present data to compare the 'metastases-free' period in the 2 groups of patients revealed no difference in the time period between primary treatment and the first appearance of metastases. Throughout the entire course of the disease, the recurrence rate in stage II carcinoma of the breast is almost identical in the 2 groups of patients (fig. 4). The 'metastases-free' interval in patients who had mastectomy alone ranged from 4 to 79 months with a median of 20 and a mean of 27.2 months. In the patients who received postoperative radiotherapy in addition to radical mastectomy, the 'metastases-free' interval ranged from 4 to 74 months with a median of 18 and a mean of 27.6 months. Whatever method of treatment was employed, over 65% of the patients were having metastases by 36 months after their primary treatment.

The survival rate of the 2 groups of patients is shown in figure 5. Although the survival rate in the group receiving only radical mastectomy is consistently better than that for patients receiving postoperative radiotherapy, the difference is not statistically significant. The results disclose that less than 35% of the patients in both groups are living at 5 years, most of them with metastases. In the entire series only 1 patient was surviving at the end of the 10 years with metastases.

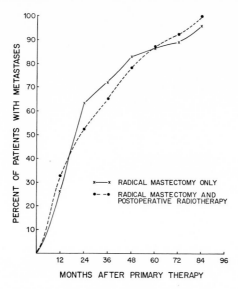

Fig. 4. Recurrence rate in patients with stage II breast cancer after radical mastectomy or radical mastectomy and postoperative radiotherapy.

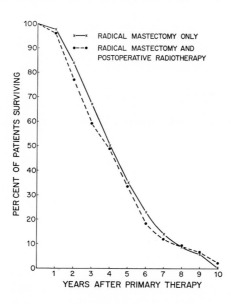

Fig. 5. Survival rate in patients with stage II breast cancer after radical mastectomy or radical mastectomy and postoperative radiotherapy.

IV. Discussion

Although this investigation is not a prospective clinical trial, the data represent a consecutive series of patients treated by surgeons and radiotherapists with essentially the same surgical procedure and radiation technique. These patients were referred to us at the outset when metastases were suspected. The inclusion of the patients in this study is based on the criteria set forth by the authors. It is doubtful that a clinical trial of the random-selection type will yield results greatly different. Although some degree of selection exists in the present study since quite evidently patients who do not develop metastases would not have been seen by us, this is not a factor biasing the results of this investigation which are in complete agreement with those from the prospective clinical trials.

The concept that carcinoma of the breast is probably a systemic disease has received both support and recognition in recent years. Local treatment, such as radical surgery or radiotherapy, does not cure breast cancer when the disease has extended beyond the local stage. If the rationale for administering postoperative radiotherapy is to destroy cancer cells in the operative sites and those already present in the regional lymph nodes, such treatment should produce a reduction in metastatic lesions in the chest wall and a decrease in incidence or delay in the appearance of metastases, thus prolonging survival. This apparently is not the case.

Results from this study clearly show that postoperative radiotherapy cannot reduce the incidence of skin recurrence, prevent distant metastases, or delay the appearance of metastases. The 'metastases-free' interval in the two groups of patients follows almost exactly the same pattern. Our data also disclose that patients with stage II breast cancer rarely survive 5 or more years free of metastases.

The recurrence rates at 18, 24, and 36 months after primary treatment in patients with positive axillary lymph nodes are 33%, 42% and 57% respectively, as reported recently by the National Surgical Adjuvant Chemotherapy Breast Cancer Study Group on a 10-year clinical trial [5]. Our results are in good agreement with the results obtained by the Surgical Adjuvant Chemotherapy

Group, of which one of the authors of the present paper (Dao) is a member. The similarity of the recurrence rate in our present study and that of the Surgical Adjuvant Chemotherapy Study further supports the validity of our present data.

Perhaps the more important findings of this study are observations pertaining to the biological nature of the breast cancer. The fact that postoperative radiotherapy was not able to prevent or reduce skin recurrence is strongly suggestive of the inability of irradiation to destroy cancer cells. In a series studied by WILLIAMS [8] of breasts removed after radiotherapy, 16 out of 17 showed cancer cells. LUMB [6] reported a study of the effect of irradiation on survival of cancer cells in 60 cases of breast cancer treated with preoperative high voltage irradiation at different dose levels. It was observed that dosages of less than 2,500 R were completely ineffective in destroying the cancer cells in the breast. Only 10% of the cases showed a 'complete absence' of evidence of malignancy in the breast when radiation doses were from 2,500 to 3,500 R. The author thus concluded that the lethal effect of X-irradiation on carcinoma cells was dependent on high dose level, which would cause excessive damage to the normal tissues. Breast cancer cells are not radiosensitive and cannot be cured by radiotherapy even if the disease is localized.

The unusual pattern of skin recurrence in patients receiving postoperative radiotherapy has been described earlier by several authors [1, 2]. The development of hundreds of dermal metastases, limited to the areas of superficial skin that had been exposed to X-irradiation, is a phenomenon that apparently is caused by the active growth of surviving cancer cells confined in an area surrounded by dense fibrosis of the skin and subcutaneous tissues as a result of irradiation. The strong barrier prevents the extension of growth beyond the boundaries of irradiation over the anterior chest wall. Extension, taking 'a path of least resistance,' often follows across the axilla to the posterior scapular region. The appearance of such patterns of skin recurrence in the irradiated patients is another example illustrating the incapability of X-irradiation to destroy cancer cells.

The significant difference in the incidence of bilateral pulmonary metastases observed as an initial sign of recurrence in the 2 treatment groups suggests that postoperative radiotherapy may indeed enhance the appearance of bilateral pulmonary metastases, possibly by effects on the 'host defense system'.

We [2] postulated earlier that survival and growth of metastases depend more on the favorable local environment than on other factors. Whether the effect of irradiation on tissues provides a favorable local environment for metastatic foci to survive and grow is not entirely clear. Later DAO and KOVARIC [1] further extended the earlier observation by an analysis of patients who received postoperative radiotherapy at Roswell Park Memorial Institute. It was also supported by experimental studies on effects of X-irradiation on 'pulmonary metastases' in rats bearing mammary cancer [3].

In the present study the frequency of metastases in the ipsilateral lung is again increased without a corresponding increase in the contralateral metastases in patients receiving postoperative radiotherapy. This observation is strongly in support of our postulation that irradiation has a local effect on the growth of metastases, possibly by producing a more favorably 'soil' for such growth.

V. Summary and Conclusion

The results following radical mastectomy (Halsted) or radical mastectomy and postoperative therapy in 176 clinical patients with stage II cancer of the breast were analyzed. All of these patients had clinical operable breast cancer but were proved to have axillary node metastases on histological examination.

The incidence of lung metastases was higher in the irradiated than non-irradiated patients. The incidence of skin recurrence in the irradiated patients was slightly lower than the non-irradiated patients. The results disclose that neither radical surgery nor combined surgery and radiotherapy can cure patients with stage II breast cancer. It appears futile to employ either radical surgery or radiotherapy in these patients. The results also demonstrate that radiotherapy in combination with radical surgery can neither prevent nor reduce skin recurrence nor delay the onset of metastases. There is, however, some evidence that the irradiation has adverse side effects on the 'host defenses' which accelerate the growth of bilateral pulmonary lesions and local effects which promote the growth of ipsilateral pulmonary metastases. The evidence is not conclusive. However, since there is no sign of benefit to the patient and some evidence of hazard, there would seem little justification for using postoperative irradiation with the radical mastectomy.

References

1. DAO, T. L. and KOVARIC, J.: Incidence of pulmonary and skin metastases in women with breast cancer who received postoperative irradiation. Surgery 52: 203–212 (1962).
2. DAO, T. L. and MOORE, G.: Clinical observation of conditions which apparently enhance malignant cell survival. Surg. Gynec. Obstet. 112: 191–195 (1961).
3. DAO, T. L. and YOGO, H.: Enhancement of pulmonary metastases by X-irradiation in rats bearing mammary cancer. Cancer 20: 2,020–2,025 (1967).
4. EASSON, E. C.: Postoperative radiotherapy in breast cancer; in FOREST and KUNKLER Prognostic factors in breast cancer, pp. 118–127 (Livingston, London 1968).
5. FISHER, B.; RAVDIN, R. G.; AUSMAN, R. K.; SLACK, N. H.; MOORE, G. E., and NOER, R. J.: Surgical adjuvant chemotherapy in cancer of the breast: Results of a decade of cooperative investigation. Ann. Surg. 168: 3 (1968).
6. LUMB, G.: Changes in carcinoma of the breast following irradiation. Brit. J. Surg. 38: 82–93 (1950).
7. PATERSON, R. and RUSSELL, M. H.: Clinical trials in malignant disease, Part III Breast cancer – evaluation of postoperative radiotherapy. J. Fact. Radiol. 10: 175–180 (1959).
8. WILLIAMS, I. G. and CUNNINGHAM, G. J.: Histological changes in irradiated carcinoma of the breast. Brit. J. Radiol. 24: 123–133 (1951).

Authors' address: Dr. THOMAS L. DAO and Dr. T. W. HSIA, Department of Breast Surgery, Roswell Park Memorial Institute, New York State Department of Health, Buffalo, NY 14203 (USA).

Discussion

Moderator:
LEONARD D. ROSENMAN, M. D., Chief, Department of Surgery, Mount Zion Hospital and Medical Center, *San Francisco, Calif.*

Discussant:
PHILIP RUBIN, M. D., Chief, Division of Radiation Therapy; Professor of Radiology, University of Rochester School of Medicine, *Rochester, N.Y.*

RUBIN: The insights that I developed in my travels to the Orient were related to learning about the various Asian religions. I'd like to recommend one book in particular, *Three Ways of Asian Wisdom* by NANCY WILSON ROSS, as a good introductory text. I now realize that the main reason for my reading this material is to develop the insight to be able to speak about the subject of breast cancer today. I would like to entitle my discussion '*The Generation Gap*,' because I feel that the people we should address ourselves to are the young people who are in the audience – the resident surgeons and radiotherapists who have heard the discussion and obviously are wondering what to do as far as their future practice pattern in the field of breast cancer.

I would like to begin with a quote concerning Hinduism, which really applies to breast cancer: 'It has often been truly said that nothing can be asserted about it that cannot also be denied.' I think this is a very appropriate comment about breast cancer. But since I'm going to address myself to the Generation Gap, I would like to use their language, and just flavor each part of the discussion with a little statement or aphorism so that we maintain perspective.

The first aphorism I'd like to offer is that *we are all against the war in Vietnam*. Now, a lot of people lose sight of this because they're more concerned with whether you're a hawk or a dove. Whether you want to bomb that country to pieces or whether you want to withdraw troops completely, the fact is that we're against the war, each in his own way, and we just want to have the war over. So all of the comments I make are addressed to the questions which have been raised; I'll allow you to draw your own conclusions as to whether you have heard hawks or doves speak to you today, but quite clearly, my comments are not going to be delivered in a personal vein. We are all against breast cancer and no matter what we say this is the personal position I want to take: we're not fighting each other, but rather breast cancer.

The second aphorism is: we should all *think Zen*. Now, I might describe to you what Zen is – it took me a little while to pick this up – Zen is 'the unique blend of Indian mysticism and Chinese naturalism sieved through a special mesh of Japanese character'... and this is the right way to think about breast cancer. The historical genesis of Zen is the Japanese way of writing the spoken Chinese word 'chan' which is a transliteration of the Sanskrit '*deeana*,' meaning 'contemplation leading to a higher state of consciousness or union with reality.' So having these three papers and getting them together last night, I was able to do quite a bit of contemplation about the subject, leading I hope to a union with reality.

I'd like to bring out a number of points, and the first point is the problem of communication. This lies in the clearness of the semantics, the choice of phrases that we all use that are designed to clarify as well as confuse. In fact, we're all trying to deliver a great deal of information. We have enough facts and figures with regard to breast cancer; however, the big problem is the concept and the way to present this.

There are two styles that we have seen material presented to us in literature. The first style is what I would call 'laissez-faire.' Everybody used different words and terms and clearly they were talking about different things. We have talked about comparing lemons and limes, but I think that one of the things that we have to recognize is that it is no longer acceptable to present data in terms of comparing treatment modalities: surgery versus surgery and radiation therapy. We have to know how these patients were selected, how they got into specified groups, and we must have some kind of a pre-treatment classification system.

We know the laws of natural selection always operate, and if there's no given reason why a patient is sent along by the surgeon for radiation therapy, usually it's because the patient has more extensive disease or a more anaplastic tumor than suspected before surgery.

The second style we use is the 'belle lettres,' the TNM classification which has been now widely accepted. This is going to be a bigger problem to solve because we're all using the same letters but it's quite clear when you begin analysing the T's that we're referring to different stages of the same cancer.

I'd like to just very briefly present a new kind of way of approaching this information, taken from FEINSTEIN's *Clinical Judgement*. I'd like to digress, and then go on to discussing the papers, because I think this approach is very relevant if we're to make progress in more accurate communication in the next decade. We can no longer count the dead and simply present survival data to one another if we're to truly understand what's going on. I call this 'Symbolic Oncotaxonomy,' which is a classification based upon symbols (fig. 1).

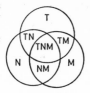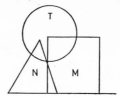

Fig. 1. Clinical spectrum of cancer staging.

I think the introduction of these Ballantine rings from beer to medicine is a very important step in outlining the clinical spectrum of cancer. If we use these Venn diagrams, you can call one 'T,' one 'N,' and one 'M' and then establish the relationships between these three categories. As you can see there are only seven clinical presentations that are possible when a patient presents with breast cancer (fig. 2).

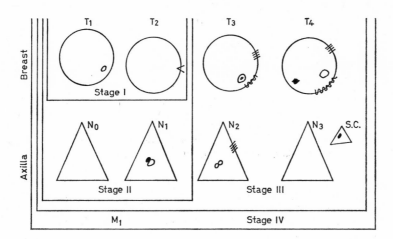

Fig. 2. Cancer paradigm: uni staging system. All stages include Paget's Disease: stage 1 = retraction or dimpling of skin; stage II = fixation to skin or chest wall; stage III = ulceration of skin; stage IV = peu d'orange.

We need a 'uni-staging' system of cancer. I feel that when we do anything by committee, and all of the international and national committees we have assigned to do this task are no exception, the end result has become an impossible system to deal with. So one of the things I'm grappling with is to develop a uni-staging system through simple symbolic diagrams. Just tune the same extent of cancer into each organ system and a uni-staging system for all cancers results. I am in the process of doing this but I won't dwell on that. Breast cancer is one of the few TNM classifications currently being used and is identical in the I.U.C.C. staging as well as the American Joint Committee of Cancer Staging.

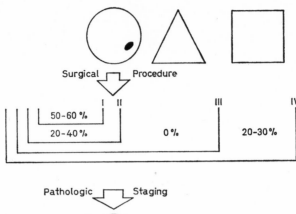

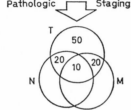

Fig. 3. Conversion ratio, clinical staging, stage I: $T_1N_0M_0$.

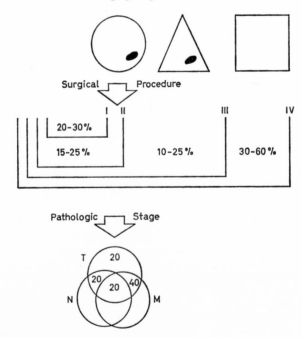

Fig. 4. Conversion ratio, Stage II: $T_1, _2N_1$.

Figure 3 is a very important concept in terms of what we're trying to do when we treat a patient.

This is Stage I breast cancer, a lesion supposedly confined to the breast, in which we're trying to identify a conversion ratio. How often is clinical Stage I cancer of the breast truly pathologic Stage I? Well, it would seem that perhaps 50–60% – this is the minimal long term survival figure – and such surviving patients are clearly limited to the breast. There's another 20–40% that involves nodes, and there's another 20–30% that probably have metastasized to distant sites. The pathologic stage is always different than the clinical presentation of the disease – and such a difference can be referred to as the 'conversion ratio.' And this ratio determines the kind of an attack that we have on the problem.

Figure 4 shows us a clinical Stage II cancer of the breast, when the nodes are involved.

In other words, this conversion ratio is the steering factor that enables us to decide what we're going to do in treatment. And remember, most of the times we're therapeutically tackling the т and N (primary and regional nodes) and we're unable to attack the metastases except with rarity.

Figure 5 shows the application of the first Venn diagram to the patterns of recurrence.

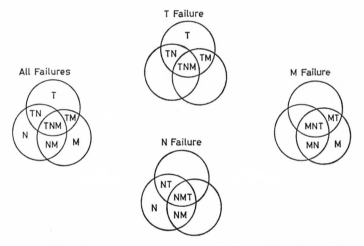

Fig. 5. Patterns of recurrences.

I think unless we know in complete detail how a patient fails, we can't identify what his problem is. There are only 7 ways a patient can fail, and if you work this out for different schemes chronologically there would be 13, i.e. TN failures versus NT. There are patients who always die because of local recurrence, even though they have nodes and metastases. This is a T failure. Another series might be of N failure; and others might be of M failures. It's important to identify specific patterns because T failures mean you need to treat the primary lesion more effectively and aggressively; and the node failures need more extensive treatment of this problem. The metastases may demand a chemotherapeutic solution. We must have information presented in this fashion; this is one of the points that Dr. FLETCHER made (fig. 6).

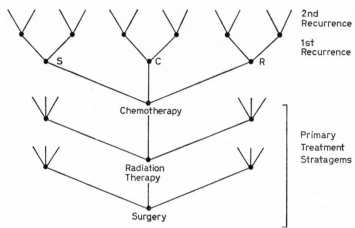

Fig. 6. Game and decision theory, game of GOPS: decision tree.

This shows the application of the Game and Decision Theory. This is the game of GOPS, what we're doing in the clinical arena. We have 3 therapeutic moves we can make, and usually there are 3 varieties of moves with each one of these moves. We have a minimum of 27 options we exercise each time we make a clinical regimen. Now unless you're aware of your options clinically, you're not free to exercise them. Many times we think we only have one or two options, but in reality we have at least 27 options, and when we undertake clinical trials we're going to block many other alternatives and this is one way of seeing the entire spectrum.

Now to go on to discussion of the papers. The third aphorism I'd like to make is *never trust the Establishment*. The 'Establishment' in this particular case is 'radical mastectomy,' the Halsted procedure. I think that Dr. FLETCHER's clinical work is impressive with particular regard to his results with preoperative irradiation. However, there are many criticisms that can be said about this report, and since he has criticized me in a similar fashion, I simply will reiterate them to him.

This is a selected and uncontrolled study. If the information is not on a controlled basis it is not valid and preoperative irradiation is unproven. Furthermore, one could even criticize the fact that he has Texas categories, and he's mixing in the TNM classification so that Stages I and II are being placed into his special categories, making the information very hard to compare with other series. However, these criticisms withstanding, the important clinical point about Dr. FLETCHER's work is the fact that the T and N (primary and nodes) are highly controlled.

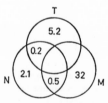

Fig. 7. FLETCHER and MONTAGUE: recurrence pattern. In the N circle, the upper segment intersected by T is for axillary nodes, the free middle segment is for supraclavicular nodes, and the lower segment is for internal mammary nodes.
Result: TN Failure 8.0;   M Failure 32.0;   Failure Index 40.0.

The measure of a sound clinician is one who knows by his experience the way to individualize treatment in a large block of patients. Taking his information: the T failures are chest wall recurrences, and the N failures are the nodal failures (axillary —0.2%, supraclavicular —2.1%, and internal mammary —0.5%). The T and N failure index, which is the addition of all the types of primary and nodal recurrences, is 8, and of course the big failure rate is due to metastatic disease. His total failure rate is 40%, and this is in the favorable categories I and II (fig. 7). We can compare this experience with the Manchester study which has been reported (fig. 8).

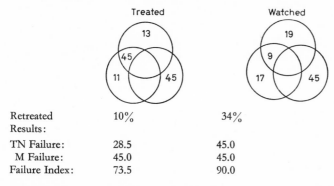

	Treated	Watched
Retreated Results:	10%	34%
TN Failure:	28.5	45.0
M Failure:	45.0	45.0
Failure Index:	73.5	90.0

Fig. 8. MANCHESTER: Recurrence pattern.

This is a treated and a watched (with regard to postoperative radiation therapy) series. Note their failure rate. And as you can see, their T and N failure rate in the treated series is much lower than the watched group. This result is the important thing to be looking at. In both instances, their local and nodal recurrence is much higher than Dr. FLETCHER's figures, and this is often lost sight of. The important thing is not only that we have more patients alive, but the quality as well as the quantity of survival shows a difference. One of the basic conflicts in the clinical investigative arena is to distinguish the difference between being a good scientist and being a good physician. I would rather be uncontrolled in Dr. FLETCHER's hands than be a control patient in Manchester, because those results whether you're 'watched' or being 'treated' clearly are not good enough. In terms of the overall results in the literature that one reads, the attitude most commonly expressed in this conference is, 'If your results are better than mine, I don't believe it... On the other hand, if your results are worse, quite clearly you've been stuck with a bunch of lemons when you should have gotten some limes for patients.' But when you look through the literature, what do you see? (Fig. 9.)

This is the real confusion in terms of breast cancer. Here are the major therapy statements – and this is why we have to look so critically at breast cancer results: these breast cancer reports condition our thinking for other cancers. And there's a habit of simply comparing surgery versus radiotherapy. There are different types of surgery, there are different types of radiation therapy, and unless we begin unscrambling this kind of information, it is absolutely impossible to have a rational discussion about therapy combinations. There is the primary lesion, there are the axillary nodes, internal mammary nodes, supraclavicular nodes, and then there's the problem of distant metastases.

The CRILE statement is for simple mastectomy only, since preservation of the regional nodes is important. Such nodes are the repository of systemic immunity to the cancer and therefore cannot be removed. However, when I asked him if he ever employed irradiation to nodes, the answer is that 44% of his patients received radiation therapy. This is clearly a

	T	N$_{AX}$	N$_{IM}$	N$_{SC}$	M	Comment
CRILE	SM	—	—	—	—	44% RT
HAAGENSEN	RM	S	—	—	—	10–15% RT
URBAN	RM	S	S	—	—	20% RT
MOORE	RM	S	C	C	C	0% RT
PETERS	T$_X$ + RT	RT	RT	RT	—	100% RT
WATSON	RM	S	RT	RT	—	70% RT
McWHIRTER	SM	RT	RT	RT	—	100% RT
FLETCHER	(RT→RM)		RT	RT	—	50–100% RT

T = Primary Target   N = Nodal   (AX = Axillary)
                                                 (IM = Internal Mammary)
                                                 (SC = Supraclavicular)
SM = Simple Mastectomy   S = Surgical Dissection
RM = Radical Mastectomy   RT = Radiation Therapy
T$_X$ = Tumorectomy   C = Chemotherapy
Comment refers to the percentage of patients in the series receiving radiation therapy.

Fig. 9. Stage I, II breast cancer; different treatment tactics.

form of McWHIRTER's technique, and this is probably why he's been able to obtain good survival figures.

HAAGENSEN is for radical mastectomy using surgical resection for the axillary nodes. However, we know he excludes at least 10–15% of his more advanced Stage I and II patients where more than the axilla is involved on triple biopsy. By careful selection, therefore, he obtains excellent results.

URBAN is a very interesting spokesman for super-radical mastectomy: he treats the primary with a radical mastectomy, then resects the axillary and internal mammary nodes. When I asked him if he ever used radiation therapy post-operatively, he answered in the affirmative. If both the axillary nodes and the internal mammary nodes are positive, he irradiates all those patients. If either one of the two is positive, he irradiates half the patients. When they're negative, surgery is a very effective technique and he doesn't send them along for radiation therapy. So here the advocate is for extended radical surgery, except that whenever nodal disease is present he also uses radiation therapy.

The MOORE hypothesis is let's go after the metastases; chemotherapy is the way to do this and as far as I know in the study they set up no radiation therapy control. I might point out some other combination techniques: PETERS, where just tumorectomy is done followed by radiation therapy; or WATSON, where radical mastectomy and a peripheral node field of radiation is done; or McWHIRTER's technique; or FLETCHER's.

The sum and substance of the literature we've had up to 1970 is this: that surgery and radiation therapy remain in balance, and that if you compare comparable groups of patients treated with logical combinations of therapy, you're going to get comparable results in every situation. This is why invariably the end result is similar. We're compensating one technique with the other technique.

In terms of McWHIRTER's position, one could say that he challenged the Establishment. The classical Halsted operation, as he said, was the undisputed method of treatment. When it was first suggested that something else should be done, it was regarded as an act of heresy. I think we can say that McWHIRTER has become part of the Establishment, now that KAAE and JOHANNSON have clearly shown that super-radical surgery versus McWHIRTER's technique in a controlled study give very comparable results.

If I have any other criticism of GILBERT FLETCHER, I might say that he has made the

Establishment, radical mastectomy, look as good as it can ever look in anybody's hands, and this shows the advantage of having a team approach in the treatment of cancer.

The important questions that Professor McWhirter raised are, 'Should lymph nodes be treated by surgery or radiation therapy, and finally how extensive a nodal area should we treat?' I think most of us agree treating the *axilla* is surgically convenient, but should we treat other surrounding nodal areas? The question as to the preference of surgery and radiation therapy is a very interesting one.

The whole subject of the lymph node barrier has to be looked at. This is totally unexplored area and only goes back about 15 years, when Ziedmann and Buss were the first ones to show that by injecting V_2 cancer cells into a peripheral lymphatic in the leg of rabbits, all these cells collected in the draining lymph node. This was proven as a valid thesis by excising the popliteal node and curing the animals. This suggested that the lymph node really was an effective barrier against systemic spead. A number of people have repeated this work; the most interesting and elegant study was published by Fisher and Fisher in 1967, using labelled red blood cells and tumor cells. They showed that most of the tumor cells were not trapped; that only those cells that were trapped seemed to really have the capacity to be clonogenic and grow, and that the failure to recover these cells suggested those that weren't trapped did not have the capacity to clone. This is evidence that biology of the cancer cell and not the lymph node barrier as it exists is not the important factor.

Now there have been a number of people who have manipulated the lymph node barrier either by surgery or irradiation, and the information here is very contradictory and inconclusive. There are a number of papers I could quote studying a number of different kinds of particle and colloid systems as well as cells. The essence of these reports is that these manipulations do tend to increase metastases, but it would seem that irradiation has a temporary effect and then the lymph node barrier is restored. Furthermore, if you believe immunity is a factor, there is another advantage in irradiation with the doses which are being used clinically, and that is the lymph nodes are restored despite irradiation and maintain both its immunologic and barrier functions.

I'd like to go on to the fourth aphorism, and that is *this is the age of overkill*. We know that we have more megatons of atomic weaponry to wipe out the populations around the globe. In an analogous way, the kind of statement that Dr. Dao has made to us is the danger of combining surgery and radiation therapy aggressively, over-treating our patients, and therefore winding up with a poorer result than we would if we utilized either one alone or neither. He has not only questioned the value of radiation therapy, but he's also questioned radical surgery.

Dr. Dao has been a major exponent in the oncology literature that radiation therapy in breast cancer may be doing some harm in patients by increasing the rate of metastases. Therefore, I've looked very hard and carefully at both Dr. Dao's present and past papers. One of the points in the current presentation that might not have been clear in the two groups that he selected is that these were patients who presented with metastases. This study is not to be equated to mean all Stage II patients who received radical mastectomy or radical mastectomy and radiation therapy. This is a selected group of these patients; these are the losers, and this is why they're all dead in ten years. I don't think the overall results for Stage II cancer are in that category. However, we all remember Dr. Dao's first statement, that the incidence of metastases was about two to three times higher in the chest wall and lung in those patients who were irradiated as compared to those who received radical mastectomy only. And although he italicized two or three times in his original paper that these two different therapeutic groups were in clinically comparable stages, the one table he had in his paper which he indicated the patients the *axilla* being negative or positive demonstrated this was not so. Ninety percent of those who had radical mastectomy and irradiation as compared to 40% of those who had radical mastectomy alone, had positive axillary nodes. This was also confirmed by Florence Chu, that if you analyse your material by therapeutic groups, you could clearly show comparing radical mastectomy versus radical mastectomy and irradiation that there was a doubling or a tripling of the incidence of metastases in chest

wall and lung. But if you broke it down by whether the individuals had positive or negative axillary nodes, it was quite clear that it didn't make any difference at all. So that the whole
basis for his original conclusion is a question of patient selection and not the type of treatment.

Again Dr. Dao in his presentation has done exactly the same thing. There is no clinical
reason that we know of why those patients went into the radical mastectomy group versus
the radical mastectomy and radiation therapy group. Appearance of metastases later does not
obviate the initial problem of selection. The reason patients were referred for radiation therapy
in the absence of randomization is that probably there was more extensive axillary disease, a
higher histologic grade of cancer, or the location of the lesion. All of these were factors
involved in the treatment selection.

Does radiation therapy really increase the incidence of breast metastases? I think that the
presentation you've made today, Dr. Dao, clearly is in part a retraction of your earlier paper.
You've quite clearly shown in this particular study that the skin metastases were lower in
those who were irradiated rather than those who had surgery alone. By contrast, you've also
shown that the pulmonary metastases are greater, but I would like to really know what you're
calling pulmonary metastases. I'm afraid some of this might be radiation reaction alone unless
all those pulmonary shadows are proven pathologically. If you want to use your figures
saying that pulmonary metastases are greater, 11% compared to 17%, the reverse can be said
of bone metastases, which you didn't present in your oral address. In other words, if you
invoke the argument that pulmonary metastases are increased, one can respond and say bone
metastases are decreased by virtue of radiation therapy. Your nodal recurrence rate has been
reduced by radiation therapy; you have a 6% proven incidence as compared to 15% when
radiation therapy was not used in this group.

The main point that you're making is that there is a difference in metastatic distribution
after irradiation, and not in incidence. Therefore, I think this requires some looking into.
There are a number of possibilities. For example, you've indicated the association of systemic
metastases with skin metastases. I think one of the important things in terms of presentation
of data in analysing mortality rates is to have more information about why we fail specifically.

This is evident in reviewing the literature. The Manchester group indicate there's no
difference in survival in surgery versus surgery and irradiation in Stages I and II, and then go
on to say more patients are dying of liver metastases in the group that received irradiation as
compared to the group that were watched. Of the patients who have died, we need to find
out all the reasons why those who were watched died. It is possible it could have been local
disease rather than metastases. So I think it's very important to indicate what the specific
reasons are for failure if we're going to try and find effective ways of combating the problem.

And I might comment finally about radiation techniques, which I find discussed in a very
disturbing manner in your paper. Dr. Dao refers to infield chest wall recurrences, and
implies that radiation therapy has been used to treat the chest wall. I see nowhere in your
paper that the chest wall was routinely treated. The radiation doses that were used we would
consider clearly less than the level that would be effective. Only 6 of the patients in this group
received supervoltage (telecobalt) radiation therapy out of about 90, in the entire series; the rest
being treated with orthovoltage therapy. It is very hard to understand exactly what the radiation
technique was, but chest wall irradiation is not mentioned and therefore I'm a little concerned
about the implication that there is a relationship between chest wall recurrence and irradiation.

And I might point out that a most important part of the relationship to skin recurrence is
also the surgery and the extent of disease. I think if metastases only appeared in the left toe after
irradiation I would really be concerned about its selectivity of site, but the reason we're treating
the chest wall is that this is the area of risk, and if one has to say where the disease would come
back most times, it's clearly in the area you're treating; otherwise you're treating the wrong area.

So rather than this being unusual to see chest wall recurrence, to me this is very usual.
This is where the disease is; you remove the disease, the wound has been seeded, we irradiate it
and we probably fail in some instances to destroy all the cancer cells. In all of the photographs, you

showed there were nodules clearly outside the treatment fields, and I think we would all agree that if you watched these patients long enough the disease indeed would spread to other areas.

Finally, and this is the important concluding note to the future generation: That is, to *be existential,* and this is from the San Francisco scene: I'm told by the hippie population that to be existential is 'not to know what will happen next,' and this is really what we mean when we're doing clinical trials. One of the hardest things to do as a physician is to randomize your patients into treatment trials and to get the information as to therapy from an envelope. I think all of us enjoy going in and telling the patient what is indicated.

The basic conflict, as I've indicated, between being an excellent clinician and being a good scientist is a major problem. It is not only showing a difference between two new methods of treatment in a controlled trial, but to show in the end that you have a better quality of T and N control and a better quantity of survivors with a new method of therapy as compared to conventional methods.

I'd just like to conclude now with a simple little statement from the Roman mythology about St. Agatha. St. Agatha is the patron saint of the breast. The story about St. Agatha goes back to antiquity, when Quintian, a man of consular dignity, tried to seduce this very lovely woman. He was quite unsuccessful, and she was sent to Aphrodisia and kept in a house of ill-repute. However, her morals would not break down despite Quintian's persistence. The governor, enraged at seeing her suffer with cheerfulness, ordered that she have her breasts shorn. Therefore she had probably the first recorded total mastectomy.

One version of the tale is that while she was dying, an earthquake came and signaled something was very, very wrong. At this point God intervened and restored her breasts. Eventually a *cultus* of St. Agatha was formed; her beatification followed, and guilds of bell founders took her for their patroness.

And what I'd like to suggest going into the 70's is that St. Agatha be the patroness of our clinical trials. I personally feel the issue of simple versus radical mastectomy is settled. The evidence indicates that radiation therapy will balance out the differences between these two surgical methods. The question is, can we save the breast as well as the woman's life? The question I'd like to put to the previous lecturers is what clinical trials are relevant in the 70's? Is tumorectomy and radiation therapy now the treatment to begin thinking about? I'd like to hear their opinions as to future trials.

If I may conclude by offering just one or two thoughts from Buddhism that I think apply: 'A man must act and live by what he has discovered to be true.' I think this is first, and the final statement is again to the resident physicians in the audience: 'Believe nothing just because you have been told it, or it is commonly believed, or because it is traditional, or because you yourself have imagined it. Do not believe what your teacher tells you merely out of respect for the teacher. But whatsoever after due examination and analysis you find to be conducive to the good, the benefit and the welfare of all beings, that doctrine believe, cling to, and take as your guide.'

FLETCHER: We did review in our material at the Anderson Hospital the location of initial metastases in the patients who had postoperative radiotherapy. And we did not find, as Dr. CHU did, any correlation at all with the size. I would say, as Dr. RUBIN, I cannot see how there can be a correlation with skin metastases when the skin has not been irradiated.

Now I would like to say a little word about tumorectomy and postoperative irradiation. Our surgeons have not yet moved into the area of doing more conservative surgery. I have had the opportunity in my travels through the world to get in contact with material which has been so treated, be it in the Curie Foundation or in England, and I have had the published data from a number of series, each amounting to perhaps a hundred or two hundred, the total amounts to about a thousand by now. Tumorectomy followed by postoperative radiotherapy has exactly the same 5 and 10 year survival rates as if you had used a radical mastectomy.

I have seen some of these women 5 to 10 years after the treatment; the palpation and the texture of the skin is hardly different – as a matter of fact the irradiated breast looks a little bit better. There are very few women who cannot stand a little bit of uplift as the years go by, and they do get that uplift by the tiny bit of fibrosis.

McWhirter: I'll try to answer Dr. Rubin's point on the question of tumorectomy. This has been done, of course; perhaps the largest series amounted to several hundred, by Moustakallio in Helsinki, and he has shown very good results with local excision of the tumor followed by radiotherapy. He published results compiled recently, I forget the actual number treated, but approximately 400–500. The results are very good, but one is able to locally excise a tumor only if it's small, and small tumors will always give good results. We have a small number of patients treated by local excision and radiotherapy, and the results are very good indeed; in fact, they're among the best of any of the methods of treatment we have. But it's a highly selected group.

An attempt to compare this with radical mastectomy in the same group of cases is being at present carried out by Hedley Atkins in London, and so far as results go there is no difference. Nor would one expect much in the way of difference because the patient suitable for local excision is not likely to have node involvement or distant metastases. The tumors must be small for the method of treatment implied.

As to developing this, as a future method of treatment, this would apply only to a limited number of breast tumors, and I've tried to make it clear in my paper that if we're going to reduce the mortality, we must seek to develop methods which will treat still more patients and offer still more patients the chance of cure.

Dao: First of all I would like to thank Dr. Rubin for his wonderful discussion and I'm not going to add anything; I don't have time to defend my data; and secondly, I don't think it's really essential. However, I wish to point out that I'm not saying that these skin recurrences developed as a result of irradiation, I'm talking about a biological phenomenon as a result of irradiation which produces a unique pattern of metastases. The lesions are in an area which was not irradiated, this I've made very clear in my paper and have also illustrated why metastases have developed into such a pattern. Clearly, irradiation of mediastinal, supra- and infra-clavicular regions caused this pattern of skin metastases. In answering Dr. Fletcher's comment, I have to make it clear that these patients were not operated on by my staff or myself. The 1962 series reported earlier was my series. The present paper deals with a series treated by surgeons and the radiotherapists outside. They are trained clinicians from different centers including ours. Through their cooperation, we've got this data together, and these were the patients who were sent to me from them when metastases were first observed. So if, as Dr. Fletcher says, these surgical results are 'atrocious', and in fact, I don't think it's too bad at all, he is intimating that these patients were 'poorly treated.' I really don't think we can do any better than these fellows outside. I want to illustrate further, especially with respect to Dr. Fletcher's comment, that even in our cooperative controlled trial series, we have very striking differences in the surgical procedures done by wellknown surgeons. For example, we studied nodal metastases from the radical mastectomy specimens from 10 to 15 university groups including ours, and we found the nodes removed ranged from zero to 100. Now to say that there are no nodes in the axilla is something hard to believe, but this can be due to the inadequate clearing of the specimen by the pathologists. On the other hand, we remove 30 to 40 nodes on an average in our patients. That's quite high. What I want to tell Dr. Fletcher is that our results are not any better than others so far as survival is concerned. I am not saying, however, that a good surgical operation is not important. I think a great deal is dependent on the stage of the disease at the time of the operation. I wish also to disagree with Dr. Rubin's suggestion that I am retracting my conclusion which I made earlier in 1962. In fact, my present data is very much in line with that of the earlier one. The pivotal point here rests upon our appraisal whether postoperative radiotherapy is beneficial to the patient. An eminent radiotherapist intimated to me recently that unless a significant reduction of mortality can be achieved by postoperative radiotherapy, any debate on the insignificant differences in the data is meaningless. I quite agree.

Front. Radiation Ther. Onc., vol. 5, pp. 231–239
(Karger, Basel/München/Paris/New York 1970)

Preoperative Irradiation with Cystectomy in the Management of Bladder Cancer

W. F. WHITMORE, Jr.

Urologic Service of the Department of Surgery, Memorial Hospital for Cancer and Allied Diseases, New York, N.Y.

In 1959 a pilot study was initiated of preoperative irradiation with cystectomy in selected patients with bladder cancer. The motivation for this study is the evidence that although either irradiation or surgery results in the five year survival of roughly similar proportions of patients with bladder tumors of corresponding stages [5], neither produces entirely satisfactory results. Furthermore, there is more or less anecdotal clinical evidence and an accumulating volume of experimental evidence to suggest that appropriate combinations of irradiation and surgery may have merit.

Materials and Methods

In characterizing the bladder tumors the MARSHALL [2] modification of the JEWETT and STRONG [1] system of staging was employed. In this system, tumors which have infiltrated no more than superficially into bladder muscle are designated as 'superficial' or 'low stage' (O, A, B,); tumors which have infiltrated deeply into muscle or through muscle into perivesical fat are designated as 'deep' or 'high stage' (B₂, C); and tumors which have invaded organs adjacent to the bladder, such as vagina, prostate, seminal vesicle or uterus, or which have invaded lymph nodes, are designated as 'metastatic' (D₁, D₂).

A preoperative clinical estimate of the stage of the tumor was derived from careful cystoscopy, biopsy and bimanual examination under anesthesia and from the adjunctive use of intravenous pyelography. Such a clinical estimate agrees with the pathologic extent of the cancer as determined by examination of the cystectomy specimen approximately 80% of the time relative to whether the tumor is of a superficial or a deep stage.

Patients were selected for cystectomy for one of two general indications: (1) Multiple low stage carcinomas, either initially too extensive for conservative treatment, or repeatedly recurrent following conservative treatment, or rapidly recurrent following conservative treatment, particularly if the lesions were of high grade either initially or subsequently. (2) High stage tumors not suitable for segmental resection, either by virtue of a history of prior tumor elsewhere in the bladder, or by reason of multiplicity, or by reason of proximity to the bladder neck. A tumor situated 2 cm or less from the bladder neck was categorically judged unsuitable for segmental resection.

Preoperative irradiation was planned for all patients in whom cystectomy was recommended excepting only those patients referred for cystectomy after failure of irradiation to control the tumor. The plan was to administer 4,000 rads in twenty fractions to the bladder and true pelvis using supervoltage irradiation in a period of four weeks and to carry out radical cystectomy between one and three months following the completion of irradiation. The irradiation was usually delivered with a cobalt 60 unit through anterior and posterior portals measuring 10×10 or 10×12 cm.

In male patients operation included excision of the bladder, prostate and seminal vesicles with enveloping fat and fascia and overlying peritoneum. In female patients the operation usually involved removal of the bladder, urethra, Fallopian tubes, ovaries, uterus and at least the anterior vaginal wall. In both sexes bilateral pelvic lymph node dissection extending from the mid-portion of the common iliac artery distally along the external iliac artery to the inguinal ligament and including the obturator, external iliac and internal iliac lymph nodes was usually a feature of the operative procedure. Excision of much of the parietal peritoneum of the pelvis made reperitonealization following this operation technically impossible.

To provide some basis for evaluation of the experience with combined irradiation and cystectomy, 145 patients subjected to radical cystectomy for bladder cancer between 1948 and 1956 but in whom prior irradiation was not employed have been analyzed and are referred to in the discussion as the 'old series' [3].

Between 1959 and 1966 radical cystectomy was advised in 327 patients with bladder cancer [4]: (1) Thirty-two patients did not receive preoperative irradiation. (2) Nine patients received other than the protocol irradiation specified above immediately prior to radical cystectomy. (3) One hundred and nine patients ('non-protocol series') had had prior irradiation for bladder cancer, usually 6,000 rads to the bladder and varying portions of the adjacent pelvis by supervoltage over a 6-to 8-week interval and usually from a few months to a year or more prior to radical cystectomy, and presented as radiation failures either with intractable urinary symptoms, or with persistent or recurrent bladder cancer, or with both. (4) One hundred and seventy-seven patients ('protocol series') received irradiation according to the protocol in anticipation of subsequent cystectomy.

The significance of any survival differences observed in the various groups of patients may be questioned on the following grounds:

1. The number of patients involved is small. Although percentages are utilized freely in presenting and discussing the data, this liberty is taken only for reasons of convenience.

2. Not only were the patients not randomized for treatment assignment after staging of the bladder cancer, but the non-irradiated control group ('old series') was not accumulated concurrently.

3. The precise causes of failure have not been analyzed in any of the treatment groups. However, the generalization may be made that approximately 80% of deaths following treatment were a result either of the treatment itself (operative mortality) or of recurrent or metastatic cancer. The incidence of local recurrences and of metastases in the different treatment groups has yet to be analyzed. The evaluation of any method of therapy of bladder cancer is dependent upon the knowledge of two distinct risks: (1) the risk of the tumor for which the immediate treatment is given and (2) the risk of development of other tumors in the bladder. In patients subjected to cystectomy for bladder cancer, the latter risk is eliminated. It is perfectly clear that radiation therapy alone has no such record of prophylaxis as far as bladder tumors are concerned but the possibility that it may reduce the rate of tumorigenesis has not been eliminated.

Operative mortality and morbidity and survival experiences are tabulated for each of three groups: (1) patients who had cystectomy only, (2) patients who had protocol irradiation with or without subsequent cystectomy, (3) patients who had non-protocol irradiation and subsequent cystectomy as radiation failures. In addition the pretreatment clinical stage of the tumor is compared to the post laparotomy ($\pm$cystectomy) pathologic stage in patients who had protocol irradiation.

Results

No significant differences in operative mortality or morbidity following radical cystectomy in the three series (table I) are apparent. The failure of preoperative irradiation, either in the protocol or non-protocol series, to produce significant variance in the expected operative mortality and morbidity following cystectomy alone does not imply that such irradiation had no adverse influences but rather that such influence was not *per se* sufficient to constitute a contraindication to such treatment. Avoiding the use of a drain in the pelvis, the gentle handling of tissues, strict attention to hemostasis and the avoidance of anastomoses in bowel or ureter wherein gross signs of irradiation are evident are some of the considerations which minimize the potentially adverse influences of irradiation. Nevertheless, some indolence in the healing of the abdominal wounds or in the resolution of pelvic wound infections was evident in the irradiated patients. Furthermore, the occasional occurrence of a mycotic aneurysm of a major pelvic artery with subsequent disruption was a usually fatal complication observed only in the patients who had received prior irradiation.

A comparison of the pre-irradiation clinical stage to the post-irradiation, post-surgical pathologic stage provides circumstantial evidence relative to the effects of the protocol irradiation on the

Table I. Bladder cancer, operative mortality and morbidity after radical cystectomy

	Old series		1959–1966 series Protocol RT		Non-protocol RT	
Deaths	16/145	11%	14/121	12%	12/81	15%
Complications	62/145	43%	52/121	43%	43/81	53%

bladder tumor (table II). The 138 patients include 121 in whom cystectomy was actually accomplished and an additional 17 in whom laparotomy revealed non-resectable tumor. In all but two instances pretreatment biopsy revealed tumor beyond the *in situ* stage and since deliberate efforts to eradicate tumor by surgical means prior to irradiation were not made, the conclusion seems justifiable that the irradiation produced a reduction in tumor stage in 26 of the 138 patients (with the two possible exceptions mentioned above). In 15 patients no residual tumor was found and in 11 patients *in situ* cancer only was found. Multiple blocks were examined from the bladders of these patients but step and serial sections were not made. Not eliminated by this analysis is the possibility that a reduction in tumor stage may have occurred in other patients as well since such a reduction might well be obscured by the normal 'error' in clinical staging. Certainly, cystoscopic observations before and after irradiation frequently indicated appreciable reduction in tumor bulk ascribable to the irradiation but for which no pathologic reductions in tumor stage were established. The theoretical capacity of irradiation to reduce the peripheral extensions of a tumor derives some support from these data.

The practical question of whether reductions in tumor stage resulting from irradiation are reflected in survival advantages is difficult to answer. Certainly, such an advantage might be obscured by the bias imposed by methods of analysis which employ the pathologic stage of the tumor *after* irradiation (and cystectomy)

Table II. Bladder cancer, comparison of preradiation clinical stage to postsurgical pathologic stage

Clinical stage		Pathologic stage				
		No tumor	*In situ*	A, B_1	B_2C	D
OAB_1	44	6	10	17	4	7
B_2C	79	9	1	15	21	33
D	15			1	5	9
Total	138	15	11	33	30	49

in calculating survival. Additional bias is introduced by the possibility of progressive tumor growth in the appreciable interval between the beginning of irradiation and cystectomy and by the fact that survival in the protocol series has been calculated from the time of cystectomy rather than from the onset of irradiation. Progressive growth of the more aggressive tumors in the interval prior to cystectomy would favor the selection of favorable cases in analyses of the pathologically low stage and high stage tumor categories following cystectomy by excluding patients whose tumors progressed to the metastatic stage in the interval. Further analyses of the data in terms of the clinical stage of the tumor immediately prior to treatment will provide circumstantial evidence concerning such possibilities.

The survival of patients who received protocol irradiation but who did not have subsequent laparotomy (or cystectomy) is given in table III. Of interest is the fact that eight of 16 patients with clinically low stage tumors survived five or more years following the completion of the protocol irradiation alone.

Table III. Bladder cancer survival of patients having irradiation only

Clinical stage		2 years		3 years		4 years		5 years	
O, A, B₁	(17)	12/17	(70%)	10/17	(58%)	9/17	(53%)	8/16	(50%)
B₂, C	(19)	9/19	(47%)	6/19	(31%)	3/19	(15%)	1/17	(6%)
D	(4)	1/4		1/4		1/4		1/4	

The survival rates for patients with low stage tumors treated by cystectomy alone, protocol irradiation followed by cystectomy, and non-protocol irradiation followed by cystectomy are shown in table IV. Also, in this table is the survival of the 15 patients in whom no residual tumor (OO) was found in the bladder following protocol irradiation and cystectomy. The 53% 5-year survival in the latter group clearly indicates that a pathologically negative bladder after irradiation (and cystectomy) provides no assurance of control of the bladder cancer. The striking feature of this tabulation, however, is the similarity in 5-year survival rates in the three different series with no survival advantage demonstrated for preoperative protocol irradiation. Furthermore, the similarity of survival rates in patients having cystectomy after a full course of irradiation had failed to control the disease, to those in patients who had cystectomy alone or protocol irradiation and cystectomy, constitutes an argument for exploring the response to irradiation before resorting to cystectomy in such patients. The latter argument, of course, disregards the possibility suggested above, that preoperative irradiation may appreciably reduce tumor stage in at least some patients.

Table IV. Bladder cancer, survival rates, pathologic stages: O, A, B_1

		2 years		3 years		4 years		5 years	
Old series (51)		37/51	(73%)	33/51	(65%)	29/51	(65%)	28/51	(55%)
Protocol series	OO (15)	14/15	(93%)	12/15	(80%)	10/15	(66%)	7/13	(53%)
	O, A, B_1 (43)	32/44	(72%)	32/44	(72%)	24/42	(57%)	20/37	(56%)
Non-protocol series (26)		17/26	(65%)	12/26	(46%)	11/26	(42%)	10/22	(45%)

In table V are shown comparable data for patients with deeply infiltrating tumors. These data suggest an improvement in survival in patients who had protocol irradiation before cystectomy, the 40% survival achieved being roughly twice that achieved in patients who had cystectomy alone. In the non-protocol group, the 30% survival achieved is better than that achieved in patients having cystectomy only. However, the non-protocol series may be regarded as a selected group of patients in the first instance because those patients who derived a good result from the irradiation would not have been included and in the second instance because patients who did poorly and died soon after irradiation would also have been excluded. In other words this group of patients includes a select portion of the radiation failures, and excludes both the best results and the poorest results of such treatment.

In table VI are shown comparable data for patients with metastatic stage neoplasms, which confirm the inadequacy of current methods of treatment of bladder cancer of this stage and indicate no benefit from the protocol irradiation.

Table V. Bladder cancer, survival rates, pathologic stages: B_2, C

	2 years	3 years	4 years	5 years
Old series (60)	17/60 (28%)	12/60 (20%)	11/60 (18%)	10/60 (17%)
Protocol series (30)	16/30 (53%)	14/30 (46%)	13/30 (43%)	12/30 (40%)
Non-protocol series (15)	6/15 (40%)	4/15 (26%)	3/15 (20%)	3/10 (30%)

Table VI. Bladder cancer, survival rates, pathologic stage: D

	2 years	3 years	4 years	5 years
Old series (34)	9/34 (26%)	5/34 (15%)	3/34 (9%)	2/34 (6%)
Protocol series (31)	3/31 (9%)	3/31 (9%)	1/31 (3%)	1/28 (3%)
Non-protocol series (29)	3/29 (10%)	1/29 (3%)	0/29	0/23

Discussion

As already pointed out, the significance of these results is made uncertain by the small numbers of patients involved and by the fact that the three major groups were not randomly nor simultaneously accumulated. On the other hand, the methods and accuracy of staging bladder cancer have not changed over the study interval and experience has demonstrated that tumor stage is the most reproducible and reliable means for categorizing patients and is the dominant determinant of prognosis [1, 3, 4]. Furthermore, the technique of cystectomy has remained the same.

Granting the effectiveness of preoperative irradiation combined with cystectomy in improving the survival of patients with deeply infiltrating cancers, how can one reconcile this observation with the failure of preoperative irradiation to improve the survival in patients with low stage cancers? Bearing in mind the theoretical curability of low stage cancers as demonstrated by the autopsy studies of Jewett and Strong and bearing in mind that most patients with low stage tumors have had one or more efforts at conservative control of their lesions before cystectomy and that such methods of conservative control may permit iatrogenic tumor dissemination, the possibility exists that irradiation fails to provide improvement in survival following cystectomy in patients with low stage tumors for the same reason that such treatment fails in patients with Stage D lesions – namely, the cancer lies outside the area of irradiation. The fact that survivals in patients with low stage tumors treated by irradiation alone or by cystectomy after the failure of irradiation are comparable to those achieved with a deliberate program of preoperative irradiation plus cystectomy is also in keeping with this speculation proposing a 'built-in' failure rate. An analysis of causes of treatment failure in these groups should yield pertinent information.

For patients with Stage D tumors, the survival prospects with or without irradiation are poor (table VI). These results are not unanticipated since the peripheral pelvic lymph nodes would not be encompassed by the radiation fields used in most of the patients in this group, even assuming that irradiation is capable of favorably influencing such lymph node metastases.

One of the problems with the reported program of therapy, even granting its effectiveness in improving the survival rate in patients with deeply-infiltrating tumors, is the duration of disability which it entails. The patient is one week in the hospital for preoperative evaluation, four weeks receiving protocol irradiation, one to three months waiting for cystectomy, at least two weeks in the hospital for cystectomy, and then a further four to eight weeks in convalescence following cystectomy. For this reason, if for no other, further exploration of programs of preoperative irradiation, designed with more practical considerations relative to time, etc. is in order.

References

1. Jewett, H. J. and Strong, G. H.: Infiltrating carcinoma of bladder: relation of depth of penetration of bladder wall to incidence of local extension and metastases. J. Urol. *55:* 366–372 (1946).
2. Marshall, V. F.: Relation of preoperative estimate to pathologic demonstration of extent of vesical neoplasms. J. Urol. *68:* 714–723 (1952).
3. Whitmore, W. F., Jr. and Marshall, V. F.: Radical total cystectomy for cancer of bladder: 230 consecutive cases 5 years later. J. Urol. *87:* 853–868 (1962).
4. Whitmore, W. F., Jr.; Grabstald, H.; Mackenzie, A. R.; Iswariah, J., and Phillips, R.: Preoperate irradiation with cystectomy; in The management of bladder cancer. Amer. J. Roentgenol. *102:* 570–576 (1968).
5. Whitmore, W. F., Jr.: The treatment of bladder tumors. Surg. Clin. N. Amer. *49:* 349–370 (1969).

Author's address: Dr. Willet F. Whitmore, Jr., Urologic Service Department of Surgery, Memorial Hospital for Cancer and Allied Diseases, *New York, NY* (USA).

Front. Radiation Ther. Onc., vol. 5, pp. 240–250
(Karger, Basel/München/Paris/New York 1970)

Combined Treatment of Non-Seminoma Testicular Cancer[1]

A Follow-Up Study

A. F. SCHROEDER, Q. CREWS, Jr. and M. B. ROTNER

Claire Zellerbach Saroni Tumor Institute of San Francisco, Mt. Zion Hospital and Medical Center, San Francisco, Calif.

In 1967 DYKHUIZEN et al. [2,5] analyzed 196 cases of testis tumors treated at the US Naval Hospital, San Diego, California. The cases were gathered over a period from 1945 to 1965. During this period several methods of treatment were employed. From 1945 to 1957, all germinal testis tumors were treated by radical orchiectomy and 260 KvP X-irradiation to the nodal stations without lymphadenectomy. Orchiectomy followed by irradiation with Cobalt-60 teletherapy was used from 1957 to 1959. In 1959 bilateral retroperitoneal lymph node resection was employed for embryonal and teratocarcinoma following full dose of 4500 rads Cobalt irradiation. This combination was rapidly discontinued after 5 of 8 patients treated in this manner had severe post-operative complications. Several patients were referred to our facility after they had undergone orchiectomy and lymphadenectomy elsewhere. They received post-operative radiation therapy only at our hospital. The current combination of pre-operative irradiation with bilateral lymphadenectomy followed by post-operative irradiation was then adopted. Currently, as in the past, all patients with pure seminoma are treated with orchiectomy and irradiation only. For purposes of this paper, our discussion will be confined to treatment of group II, III, and IV carcinoma.

Germinal tumors of the testis were classified as:

Group I   Pure seminoma
Group II   Embryonal carcinoma pure or with seminoma

[1] The opinions or assertations contained herein are the private ones of the authors and not to be construed as official nor as reflecting the views of the Navy Department, or the Naval Service at large.

Group III   Teratocarcinoma pure or with seminoma
Group IV   Teratocarcinoma with embryonal carcinoma or
                  choriocarcinoma with or without seminoma
Group V   Choriocarcinoma

Patients were clinically staged as follows:

Stage I   Localized to the testis without evidence of
             spread to the capsule or cord structures
Stage II   Spread to the capsule or spermatic cord or
             regional lymph nodes, unilateral or bilateral,
             pelvic or periaortic
Stage III   Spread above the diaphragm or distant metastases

Treatment Techniques

Following orchiectomy the patients with stage I disease and those deemed operable in stage II were treated with Cobalt-60 teletherapy. Abdominal bath with shielding of the iliac crests and proximal femora was initiated (fig. 1). All patients were treated with opposed fields at 150 rads per fraction, 5 fractions per week (750 rads/week) to a total of 2250 rads in 3 weeks. Within 3–10 days, the patients underwent a bilateral retroperitoneal lymph node dissection. The dissection was carried down to the bifurcation of the aorta on each side.

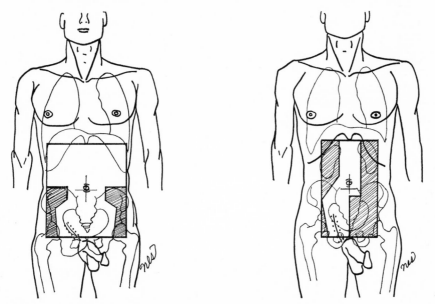

Fig. 1. Initial fields of irradiation, opposed total abdomen and pelvis.
Fig. 2. Post operative, opposed, constricted, periaortic and pelvic fields.

A chevron or bilateral subcostal incision was made, affording excellent exposure of the nodal bed. Following recovery from surgery, usually 2 weeks, the patients returned to the therapy department for an additional 2250 rads to constricted fields encompassing the periaortic and pelvic nodes (fig. 2). The same fractionation scheme was used and the total tumor dose carried to 4500 rads. If the capsule or cord structures were involved, the hemiscrotum was included in the field. If the patient had had previous orchiopexy and/or the capsule or cord structures were involved, the inguinal nodes were included in the field (fig. 3).

Depending upon the hematopoietic picture, the patients were placed on a 1–3 week rest and then received 4000 rads to the mediastinum and bilateral supraclavicular nodes (fig. 4). This tumor dose was also delivered at the rate of 150 rads per fraction, 750 rads per week.

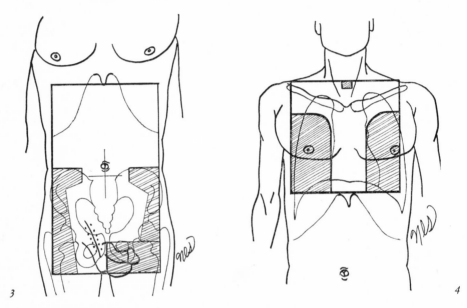

Fig. 3. Opposed fields of total abdomen, pelvis, and hemiscrotum.
Fig. 4. Opposed mediastinum and bilateral supraclavicular fields.

Previous techniques had numerous major complications, such as wound dehiscence, bowel fistulae, intestinal obstruction, and peptic ulcer. With the present technique, nausea and vomiting often occurred, but was controlled with either Compazine, 10 mg t.i.d., or Torecan, 10 mg t.i.d. Patients had reduction of peripheral blood elements during treatment, but none was persistant or prevented completion of treatment. There were no major complications and no operative mortality.

A total of 230 patients were evaluated with 234 tumors as 4 patients had second primaries. There were 82 patients with pure seminoma, 14 seminoma with embryonal elements, 2 seminoma with teratocarcinoma elements, and one had seminoma with choriocarcinoma elements.

Pure teratocarcinoma occurred in 29 patients, teratocarcinoma with embryonal elements 14, teratocarcinoma with choriocarcinoma elements 3.

Pure embryonal carcinoma presented in 46 patients, embryonal cell with teratocarcinoma 3, and 4 had embryonal with choriocarcinoma elements.

There were 7 patients with pure choriocarcinoma. Also 6 patients had pure teratoma. An additional 9 patients presented with either rhabdomyosarcoma, reticulum cell sarcoma, adenocarcinoma, fibrosarcoma, dysgerminoma, androblastoma, or undifferentiated carcinoma. One patient had a tumor with histologic type not designated. See table I.

Table I. Testicular tumors 1945–1969 Total patients – 230

Seminoma		Choriocarcinoma	7
Pure	82	Teratoma	6
With embryonal	14	Others	9
With terato CA	2	Androblastoma	1
With Chorio	1	Dysgerminoma	3
Embryonal		Fibrosarcoma	1
Pure	46	Reticulum cell sarcoma	1
With terato CA	3	Rhabdomyosarcoma	1
With chorio	4	Adenocarcinoma	1
Terato CA		Undifferentiated	1
Pure	29	Type not designated	1
With embryonal	14		
With chorio	3		

Results

In the reports of DYKHUIZEN *et al.* [2] and KUROHARA *et al.* [5], 6 patients had been treated with orchiectomy followed by Cobalt-60 teletherapy alone at the Naval Hospital, San Diego, CA. All six of these patients were alive without disease at 5 years and continue to do well, 100% 5-year survival.

From 1948 to 1965, 21 patients were treated with lymphadenectomy plus post-operative Cobalt-60 alone. Two patients are lost to follow up and must be considered dead. Records are inadequate during this period of time to determine the number of patients with positive nodes and negative nodes. Twelve of these 21 patients are free of disease, 57% 5-year survival (table II).

Nine patients were treated with lymphadenectomy plus post-operative Cobalt-60 since 1965. Four had positive nodes and 1 of these 4 is alive without disease at 2 years, 25%. Five patients had negative nodes and 4 of these 5 are alive without disease at 2 years, 80%. Overall survival 56%. The figures for the two periods related to each other very closely (table III).

From 1948 to 1965, patients who had pre-operative Cobalt-60 plus lymphadenectomy plus post-operative Cobalt had a combined 5-year survival without disease of 79%. With positive nodes the survival without disease was 33% and with negative nodes 100% (table IV).

Table II. Lymphadenectomy – post-operative Cobalt-60 1948–1965, total patients – 21[1]
(2 lost to follow-up)

No. of patients	5-year survival without disease
19	12 (12/19) 63%
21 (lost = dead)	12 (12/21) 57%

[1] Records inadequate to determine number with positive nodes vs. negative nodes.

Table III. Lymphadenectomy – post-operative Cobalt-60 Since 1965, total patients – 9

	No. of patients	2-year survival without disease
Positive nodes	4	1 (1/4) 25%
Negative nodes	5	4 (4/5) 80%
Total patients	9	5 (5/9) 56%

Table IV. Cobalt-60 – Lymphadenectomy – Cobalt-60 1948–1965, total patients – 19

	No. of patients	5-year survival without disease
Positive nodes	6	2 (2/6) 33%
Negative nodes	13	13 (13/13) 100%
Total patients	19	15 (15/19) 79%

Since 1965, an additional 9 patients treated by this combined technique are eligible for evaluation of 2-year survival. Of these patients, 8 had negative nodes and 1 had positive nodes. Of the 8 with negative nodes, 6 are alive without disease. The one with positive nodes is alive without disease (table V).

Therefore, 28 cases of testis carcinoma, group II, III, and IV treated with Cobalt-60 teletherapy, lymphadenectomy and post-operative irradiation are eligible for survival from 2 years to 10 years. There are 43% with positive nodes alive without disease and 90% with negative nodes without disease, with an overall of 79% (table VI).

Table V. Cobalt–60 – Lymphadenectomy – Cobalt-60 Since 1965, total patients – 9

	No. of patients	2-year survival without disease		
Positive nodes	1	1	(1/1)	100%
Negative nodes	8[1]	6	(6/8)	75%
Total patients	9	7	(7/9)	78%

[1] Two patients developed pulmonary metastases.

Table VI. Cobalt–60 – Lymphadenectomy – Cobalt-60 Overall 1948–1969, total patients – 28

	No. of patients	2-year survival without disease		
Positive nodes	7	3	(3/7)	43%
Negative nodes	21	19	(19/21)	90%
Total patients	28	22	(22/28)	79%

Discussion

For years there has been little argument against the treatment of seminoma with orchiectomy and irradiation only [3]. The radio-sensitivity of the tumor is high, the dose necessary to irradiate the tumor low, and the 'cure' rates high. Initially the results of treatment of teratocarcinoma and embryonal cell carcinoma with irradiation were low [3]. It was postulated, therefore, that radiation therapy was not effective alone in controlling the latter two types of testicular tumor. Following World War II lymphadenectomy gained popularity in the treatment of these carcinomas [12].

It was also thought that pre-operative irradiation would decrease the risk of spread of tumor cells at the time of surgery as the cells would be less capable of reproduction and growth and that the host bed would be less suitable for the cells. The tumor would also have better oxygenation with an intact blood supply. It was also possible that some tumors would be made resectable under the influence of the irradiation.

The original treatment of full course irradiation plus lymphadenectomy was fraught with many complications and discontinued. The rationale of pre-operative irradiation still prevailed and pre and post-operative irradiation was combined with lymphadenectomy. LOWRY et al. [7], THOMAS and BISCHOFF [16], LEADBETTER [6] and McKEIL [10] had reported several cases of bilateral nodes and JAMIESON and DOBSON [4] had described cross communication of lymphatic drainage of the testis. Therefore, it was elected to perform bilateral lymphadenectomies as recommended by STAUBITZ [16]. MAIER et al. [9], showed the same survival rates with similarly staged tumor, positive and negative nodes with unilateral versus bilateral lymphadenectomies. GEORGE [2] chose an abdominal bath, as he felt if nodes were choked with tumor, there could be collateral spread of the disease outside of the routine periaortic fields. He also thought if there were collections of small numbers of cells in areas such as the liver, perhaps low dose pre-operative irradiation could destroy them.

In the early work at the US Naval Hospital, San Diego, CA, the majority of recurrence was in the mediastinum and lungs. This was noted by NOTTER and RANUDD [11] and SANDEMAN [13] even when clinical and surgical studies failed to show abdominal positive nodes. SAYEGH et al. [14] demonstrated direct lymphatic connection between the lymphatics of the testis and mediastinal nodes which by-passed the nodal stations at the renal hilum. Hence, it was elected to prophylactically treat the mediastinum and supraclavicular fossae. It is noted that CASTRO [1] failed to demonstrate any benefit from treating the mediastinum and supraclavicular fossae in the study at M. D. Anderson Hospital.

One cannot discount the fact that 6 patients in our study were treated with Cobalt teletherapy alone and are alive without disease. In our study, 25% of the cases had positive nodes and this percentage or greater is quoted by others. Considering this, perhaps 1 or 2 of the patients had positive nodes that were controlled with irradiation.

It is noted that the cases in our study that had lymphadenectomy followed with full dose Cobalt-60 teletherapy did not provide a comparative survival rate with the 'sandwich' technique. Both the groups treated from 1948–1965 (overall survival 57%) and the group since 1965 (overall survival 56%) did not compare with the 79% survival with the Cobalt-lymphadenectomy-Cobalt technique.

There are proponents, MacKay and Sellers [8] for radiation therapy alone, for lymphadenectomy, Staubitz and Whitmore [15, 17] and combined radiation therapy and lymphadenectomy, Dykhuizen and George [2]. The only way to decide the true worth of each modality is a randomized series, such as has been developed at Walter Reed US Army Hospital.

Acknowledgement

The authors gratefully acknowledge the assistance of: Norman L. Swensson, Cdr., M.C., USN, US Naval Hospital, San Diego, CA, Medical Illustrator; and Robert Easter, Medical Photographer; Miss Hiroko Kowta, Technical Assistance; and Miss Roberta Sitzman, Secretary, Claire Zellerbach Saroni Tumor Institute of San Francisco.

Summary

The various techniques used since 1945 at the US Naval Hospital, San Diego, California, for the treatment of non-seminoma germinal tumors of the testis are described. Six patients have been treated with orchiectomy followed by Cobalt-60 teletherapy alone, and all 6 are alive at least 5 years post-therapy. Twenty-one patients were treated with lymphadenectomy plus post-operative Cobalt-60 from 1948–1965 with a 5-year survival of 57%, and 9 patients were treated in a similar fashion since 1965. In 1959 a combination of pre-operative Cobalt-60 teletherapy, lymphadenectomy, and post-operative Cobalt-60 was developed. Since that time, 28 patients have been treated in this manner. Three of 7 or 43% with positive nodes are alive at 2 years, without evidence of disease. Nineteen of 21 or 90% with negative nodes are alive at 2 years, without evidence of disease. Nineteen of 21 or 90% with negative nodes are alive at 2 years without evidence of disease. An overall of 22 of 28 or 79% survival has been achieved.

References

1. CASTRO, J. R.: Lymphadenectomy and radiation therapy in malignant tumors of the testicle other than pure seminoma. Cancer *24:* 87–91 (1969).
2. DYKHUIZEN, R. F.; GEORGE, F. W.; KUROHARA, S.; ROTNER, M.; SARGENT, C. R. and VARNEY, J. K.: The use of Cobalt-60 teletherapy or X-ray therapy with and without lymphadenectomy in the treatment of testis, germinal tumors: a 20 comparative study. J. Urol. *100:* 321–328 (1968).
3. FRIEDMAN, M. and DI RIENZO, A. J.: Treatment of trophocarcinoma (embryonal carcinoma) of the testis. J. Radiol. *80:* 550–565 (1963).
4. JAMIESON, J. K. and DOBSON, J. F.: The lymphatics of the testicle. Lancet *1:* 493 (1910).
5. KUROHARA, S. S.; GEORGE, F. W.; DYKHUIZEN, R. F. and LEARY, K. I.: Testicular tumors, analysis of 196 cases treated at the US Naval Hospital in San Diego. Cancer *20:* 1089–1098 (1967).
6. LEADBETTER, W. F.: Treatment of testis tumors based on their pathological behavior. J. amer. med. Ass. *151:* 275–280 (1953).
7. LOWRY, E. C.; BEARD, D. E.; HEWITT, L. W. and BARNER, J. L.: Tumors of the testicle: analysis of one hundred cases: a preliminary report. J. Urol. *55:* 373 (1946).
8. MACKAY, E. N. and SELLERS, A. H.: A statistical review of malignant testicular tumors based on the experience of the Ontario Cancer Foundation Clinics, 1938–1961. Canad. med. Ass. J. *94:* 889–899 (1966).
9. MAIER, J. G.; BUSKIRK, K.; SULAK, M.; PERRY, R. H. and SCHAMBER, D. T.: Anvaluation of lymphadenectomy in the treatment of malignant testicular germ cell neoplasm. J. Urol. *101:* 356–359 (1969).
10. MCKIEL, C. F.: Surgery of testicular tumors. Surg. Clin. N. Amer. *49:* 99–103 (1969).
11. NOTTER, G. and RANUDD, N. E.: Treatment of malignant testicular tumors: a report on 355 patients. Acta radiol. *2:* 134–151 (1964).
12. PATTON, J. F.; SEITZMAN, D. N. and ZONE, R. A.: Diagnosis and treatment of testicular tumors. Amer. J. Surg. *99:* 525–532 (1960).
13. SANDEMAN, T. F.: Testicular tumors. J. Coll. Radiol. Austr. *8:* 134–151 (1964).
14. SAYEGH, E.; BROOKS, T.; SACHER, E. and BUSCH, F.: Lymphangiography of the retroperitoneal lymph nodes through the inguinal route. J. Urol. *95:* 102–107 (1966).
15. STAUBITZ, W. J.; MAGOSS, I. V.; GRACE, J. T. and SCHENK, W. G.: Surgical management of testis tumors. J. Urol. *101:* 350–355 (1969).
16. THOMAS, G. J. and BISCHOFF, A. J.: Tumors of the testis: analysis of 80 cases. J. Urol. *72:* 41 (1954).
17. WHITMORE, W. F.: Some experiences with retroperitoneal lymph node dissection and chemotherapy in the management of testis neoplasms. Brit. J. Urol. *34:* 436–447 (1962).

Authors' addresses: Dr. ALAN F. SCHROEDER, Claire Zellerbach Saroni Tumor Institute of San Francisco, Mt. Zion Hospital and Medical Center, *San Francisco, CA*; Dr. QUINTOUS CREWS, Jr., Head Radiation Therapy, US Naval Hospital, *San Diego, CA*; Dr. MELVIN B. ROTNER, Urology Department, US Naval Hospital, *San Diego, CA* (USA).

Discussion

Moderator:
JUSTIN J. STEIN, M. D., Professor of Radiology; Chief, Division of Radiation Therapy; Director, Cancer Research Institute, UCLA Center for Health Sciences, *Los Angeles, Calif.*

Discussant:
JOSEPH J. KAUFMAN, M. D., Professor, Department of Surgery, Division of Urology, UCLA Center for Health Sciences, *Los Angeles, Calif.*

KAUFMAN: About 6 or 7 years ago, Dr. STEIN and I at UCLA became interested in the treatment of bladder tumors with preoperative irradiation and 5-fluorouracil. I though I would bring you up to date on some of the results because they dovetail with the statements made by Dr. WHITMORE today. We were disenchanted with large doses of radiation therapy before surgery because we were confronted with the same unacceptable morbidity and mortality alluded to by Dr. WHITMORE in regard to cystectomy in patients who had been heavily irradiated preoperatively. We had the idea at that time that perhaps 5-fluorouracil and cobalt teletherapy might be synergistic in their action, that we could reduce the dosage of cobalt-60 in these patients to a 3,500 rad level preoperatively and perhaps achieve the same sterilization affect and betterment of long term results following subsequent cystectomy that had been achieved with the use of high doses of preoperative radiation therapy.

We had 33 patients in stages A and B_1 categories. It is notable that no tumor was found in the specimen in 16 of 33, or 48%. This figure is important in later discussion. All of the new patients were sent to us for cystectomy because of the rapid rate of tumor recurrence, the patients having obviously escaped more conservative measures. Nine of these patients subsequently died of tumor. Not a really outstanding result, but it is interesting that in this group of patients there were 12 in whom cystectomy was avoided. Twelve patients in this group among the 3 year survivors are still free of tumor or have had tumors which became easily manageable by transurethral electroresection. In the B_2 and C lesions, tumors that infiltrate deeply, we do not have such a happy story. We found no tumor, however, in the specimen after combined radiation and chemotherapy in 8 patients out of 21. It is of interest that 4 of these patients escaped cystectomy initially but 4 patients of these 8 subsequently died of disseminated carcinoma. Forty-four per cent were alive 3 years and 36% were alive at 4 years.

Comparing our results with Dr. WHITMORE's in Stage A and B_1 tumors, he found 36% down-staging and in this group we found 46% down-staging. Whitmore reports 14% whose bladders were sterilized of tumor as a result of preoperative radiotherapy; we had 48% that were freed of tumor. Nonetheless our 4 year survivals are not quite as good as Dr. WHITMORE's. I doubt that the differences are statistically significant. Furthermore, WHITMORE included stage 0 in his series and we have no stage 0 cases. We had 12 patients who escaped cystectomy in our series and perhaps this is a real advantage of the combined 5-fluorouracil and cobalt teletherapy in contradistinction to the radiotherapy alone.

In the B_2 and C tumors at 3 years the figures reported by WHITMORE and by our group are 26% and 40% respectively. We found 38% who had no tumors following the combined radio-therapy-chemotherapy compared to Dr. WHITMORE's 11 per cent, and downstaging we felt existed in 76% compared to his 16%. We all use Dr. WHITMORE's results as standards for measuring our results for two reasons: he is in a cancer hospital, he is an expert urological surgeon. We have to assume that Dr. WHITMORE is getting the optimal results from radiation therapy and surgery. We now feel that our own combination of therapy perhaps has no advantage over 4,000 rads of preoperative radiotherapy, but perhaps it has merit in the treatment of superficial carcinomas that are recurring rapidly.

In regard to testis tumors we have recently reviewed our results with 65 patients at UCLA followed for a minimum of 5 years after radical retroperitoneal lymph node dissection. The 5 year survival in our group was 82% for the stage A and B tumors (i.e. those tumors which have confined themselves to the testis or have spread only to adjacent structures or to the retroperitoneal lymph nodes). Dr. SCHROEDER claims a 90% 2–10 year survivorship in patients with stage A tumors making a case perhaps for the 'sandwich' treatment, but with post lymphadenectomy irradiation the results are comparable. Dr. SCHROEDER, I would say that there must be some theoretical merit in using preoperative radiotherapy, but I would like to see more assurance that what we are really irradiating are positive nodes. We all know the methods we have available of knowing whether positive nodes exist. The intravenous urogram may show deviation of the ureters or change of axis of the kidney. Lymphangiography may reveal positive nodes. However, many nodes that are occupied by tumor do not show up in the lymphangiogram and therefore there is no way of knowing accurately whether positive nodes exist on this basis. Therefore we have more or less abandoned lymphangiography except in the study of seminoma. We use the vena cavogram frequently in the study of patients with carcinoma of the testis. I would like to bring your attention to a method of determining whether there are nodes in the retroperitoneal area without recourse to some of these radiographic techniques, that is the use by the urologist of a peritoneotomy through the inguinal incision at the time of the orchiectomy. The urologist can easily place his hand in the peritoneal cavity and palpate the retroperitoneal structures as high as the renal pedicles. This merely requires splitting the internal oblique muscles and opening the peritoneum. It does not add to the morbidity of the orchiectomy, which in any case should be done through a generous inguinal incision in order to remove the entire spermatic cord. With knowledge of positive retroperitoneal nodes in advance, perhaps we would be doing a greater service to patients to give them irradiation therapy preoperatively.

I would like to ask Dr. SCHROEDER if he has seen radiation nephritis in these cases; it seems to me that his abdominal bath and dosage of radiation therapy come close to what would constitute serious nephrotoxic radiation effects.

In conclusion we really do not know the place of radiation therapy in the treatment of carcinoma of the bladder, nor do we know the place of radiation therapy plus cystectomy. We are still pretty much in limbo. The results are good for testicular tumor, no matter what is done, as long as one employs lymphadenectomy and radiation therapy, either after surgery or before *and* after the operation.

SCHROEDER: To answer your question, Dr. KAUFMAN, in regard to the number of patients with positive nodes, and why the decreased survival rate in this group. In reviewing the original articles, some cases included in this group were those that had had lymphadenectomy and then a full course of post operative irradiation. This would account for the difference in our data and that presented by DYKHUIZEN. In the current 28 cases, there were only 7 with positive nodes. With the passing of time, the survival rate has decreased.

In regard to complications: To my knowledge we have not had any radiation nephritis. According to the work of LUXTON and KUNKLER, the radiation tolerance of the kidneys is approximately 2,300 rads at 1,000 rads per week. Other people think that this may be 2,500 rads or greater. Our dose of 2,250 rads to the abdomen was in a range that we felt with the added internal scatter and transmission through our blocks that we were within tolerance. We have not had any major problems with liver. There is a recent article by KUROHARA in regard to the effects of our treatment technique with liver.

ROSWIT: Stanford takes the same cases of bladder cancer, Stages A–C, and salvages one-third of them with irradiation alone. WHITMORE with 4,000 rads and total cystectomy has a 36% survival. And now you fellows from UCLA come along and throw in 5 F–U. Why don't you do all three?

Front. Radiation Ther. Onc., vol. 5, pp. 251–261
(Karger, Basel/München/Paris/New York 1970)

Recent Trends in the Management of Advanced Ovarian Carcinoma

R. T. L. LONG
Ellis Fischel State Cancer Hospital

Carcinoma of the ovary is a formidable lesion. It remains relatively silent in its early growth, with symptoms usually resulting from abdominal enlargement by cystic tumor masses or peritoneal tumor seeding with ascites, or from invasion and compression of adjacent viscera. Additional problems arise because of the difficulty in obtaining a biopsy and making an accurate diagnosis prior to laparotomy, the inadequate lateral and posterior exposure obtained within the pelvis, and the frequent involvement of adjacent viscera not ordinarily included in conventional removal of the female pelvic viscera. Ovarian carcinoma appears first in the third decade, with the exception of malignant teratoma of childhood, and rises to a peak incidence in the sixth decade. Overall survival rates vary from 10% to 20% [3, 8].

Classification

Staging. Of all anatomic and histologic criteria, staging is the most important in predicting survival [8, 16]. Staging based on operability is not of great value, since it does not allow comparison of extent of lesions with accuracy, and may vary from surgeon to surgeon. Staging based on exact anatomical extent of tumor as determined at laparotomy, however, is of great prognostic value. A conservative outline is given here.

Stage I – tumor confined to one or both ovaries.
Stage II – spread beyond the ovarian capsule, but confined to uterus, broad ligaments, or tubes.

Stage III – those with spread to adjacent peritoneum, rectum, bladder, small bowel or
        omentum, but still within limits of the greater pelvis.
Stage IV - metastases to upper abdomen or distant sites.

Examination of the distribution by stage reveals 85% of cases
to occur in Stages III and IV, with 15% of cases in the early stages.
Stage III (locally advanced) lesions comprise 25% of the total. The
excellent survival of Stage I and II lesions is significant compared
with the poor survival of the advanced lesions (fig. 1). Stage I
lesions have been treated primarily by surgery, and the extent
beyond oophorectomy seems to have little significance. The mode
of treatment (combinations of therapy) seems to have its greatest
significance in the management of locally advanced lesions.

Although the presence of ascites is a grave sign, it does not
denote a hopeless prognosis. At the Ellis Fischel Hospital, these
patients had a 6.6% five-year survival. If the ascites is mucinous,
the outlook is much more favorable.

Histology. Histological variation has the same significance as
tumor grading. A simple classification is outlined below.

1. Tumors derived from the Graafian follicle. (a) Granulosa cell – low grade malignancy.
(b) Theca cell- usually benign.

2. Tumors derived from the early mesenchyme. Dysgerminoma – malignant.

3. Tumors related to early developmental stages of the male gonad. (a) Arrhenoblastoma-
low grade malignancy. (b) Virilizing lipoid cell – benign and malignant variants. (c) Hilus
cell – very little malignant potential.

4. Tumors arising from totipotent anlage. (a) Adult teratoma – usually occurs as classical
dermoid cyst, malignant variant is epidermoid carcinoma. (b) Embryonal teratoma – usually
highly malignant, occurs in childhood. (c) Embryonal carcinoma – epithelial malignant
variant of (b).

5. Tumors arising from fibrous stroma. (a) Fibrosarcoma – firm, of low malignant
potential. (b) Sarcoma, unclassified – soft, highly malignant.

6. Tumors arising from embryonal structures related to the ovary. (a) Brenner tumor –
small, solid, benign. (b) Endosalpingioma – resembles tubal epithelium, regress following
oophorectomy. (c) Serous papillary carcinoma – presumed to be derived from tubular epithelium, this is the most common variant of malignant ovarian tumors. Its distinguishing
characteristic is the gross papillary, grape or cauliflowerlike mass. Care should be taken to
distinguish these lesions from the true mucinous tumors, which occasionally develop a low
grade papillary structure. (d) Mucinous or 'pseudomucinous' tumors – presumably derived
from enteric anlage. They consist of innumerable daughter cysts within progressively larger
cysts, each filled with gelatinous mucin, lined by columnar epithelium. Despite the benign
appearance, they are capable of implanting extensively on the peritoneal surfaces, producing
the condition known as pseudomyxoma peritonei.

Tumor histology exerts a lesser influence on survival than does
staging, this influence being due in part to the marked correlation
between high stage and high grade tumors. The undifferentiated
and solid adenocarcinomas, in our experience, have been virtually

all Stage III or Stage IV lesions [8]. Granulosa tumors, however, occur with 60% of cases in Stages I and II. Mucinous carcinomas have approximately one-fourth of cases in early stages, while papillary carcinoma occurs in these stages in only 10% of patients. There is little difference in survival between the three most common tumors- papillary, mucinous, and solid adenocarcinoma. With undifferentiated carcinoma, survival is very poor. Granulosa carcinoma appears to be a favorable type (fig. 2).

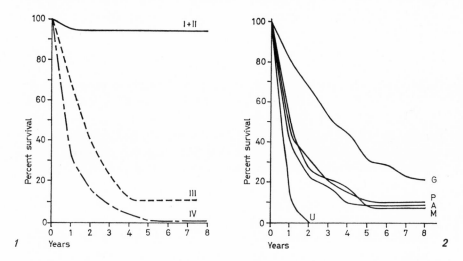

Fig. 1. Accumulative survival of determinate cases of ovarian carcinoma by stage. Stage I – 18 patients; Stage II – 4 patients; Stage III – 35 patients; Stage IV – 89 patients.
Fig. 2. Accumulative survival by histologic type of tumor. The better survival of tumor types which have greater numbers in the early stages demonstrates the difficulty in separating the effect of tumor type and tumor stage on survival. G=granulosa carcinoma; P = papillary carcinoma; A = solid adenocarcinoma; M = mucinous carcinoma; U = undifferentiated carcinoma.

Treatment

Although surgical excision remains the mainstay of therapy, adjunctive treatment with radiotherapy contributes greatly to success. Chemotherapy with alkylating agents, and more recently, hormonal therapy has taken a place in the treatment of these primary gonadal lesions [6, 9]. The combinations, and sequence of modalities should be based on the stage of the lesion and on its histology.

Surgery. The most effective treatment of these lesions is surgical. For tumors confined to the ovary, simple oophorectomy may be adequate. This is based on the experience at the Ellis Fischel Hospital in which 9 patients with Stage I disease were treated by oophorectomy and another 9 by 'panhysterectomy'. All patients survived free of disease except one patient in whom the cyst was ruptured at laparotomy. BARNES [2] found 90 patients reported in the literature with carcinoma confined to one ovary, who were treated by unilateral oophorectomy, and 95 similar patients treated by radical surgery. There was no statistical difference in survival. Thus, if childbearing is an important consideration, a precedent for conservative surgery has been established. However, when the contralateral ovary appears normal, it will contain metastases in 17% of cases [2]. Because of this, and the occasional occurrence of endometrial metastases, we recommend removal of both ovaries, tubes, and the uterus. The pelvic peritoneum and omentum should also be excised widely because these are frequent sites of occult implantation. Frozen section diagnosis is mandatory to establish the nature of the tumor at the time of laparotomy.

Only a small percentage of patients will have tumors limited to the ovary. The vast majority will have advanced lesions. In this circumstance, if the tumor is confined to the greater pelvis, despite involvement of adjacent viscera, including bowel, the chance for ultimate control may be good, if the patient is subjected to irradiation, followed by a well conceived excision of all sites of extension. As illustrated in figure 3, the survival rate after radical surgical resection (varying from panhysterectomy to pelvic exenteration) was best if combined with radiotherapy. If no adjunctive irradiation was used, survival was much poorer. Oophorectomy with radiotherapy provided some survivors beyond the fifth, but not the seventh year. Radiotherapy alone, or oophorectomy alone for these locally advanced lesions provided no long term survivors.

Figure 4 is a study of the effect of adjunctive radiotherapy on radical resection of Stage III ovarian cancers. The operative procedures varied from patient to patient, each procedure tailored by the surgeon to remove the local extensions of the tumor. The most commonly employed procedure was wide hysterectomy with

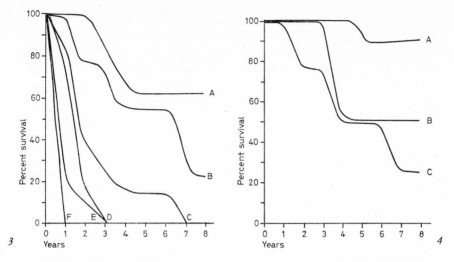

Fig. 3. Effect of various treatment regimens on survival of patients with Stage III carcinoma. A = radical surgery with radiotherapy; B = radical surgery without radiotherapy; C = oophorectomy with radiotherapy; D = oophorectomy alone; E = no treatment; F = radiotherapy alone.

Fig. 4. Survival after various combinations of radical surgery and radiotherapy. A = preoperative irradiation followed by radical surgery (8 patients); B = radical surgery followed by external irradiation (4 patients); C = radical surgery without irradiation (4 patients).

salpingo-oophorectomy, combined with anterior resection of the rectum. Survival was much enhanced by adjunctive irradiation, and this was apparently more effective if given preoperatively. Approximately half of these patients were treated with 240 kV equipment, and the remainder with Co-60. At present we are treating these patients with Cobalt to 4,500 rads through two anterior and posterior ports extending to the level of the umbilicus, and delivering 200 rads daily.

The operation for Stage III lesions is best carried out six weeks following radiotherapy, when regression of the tumor mass appears to have reached a maximum. In a typical situation, the omentum, terminal small bowel and cecum, and rectosigmoid will be adherent to the pelvic tumor mass. The attachment of the omentum to the stomach and colon is transsected, allowing it to fall into the pelvis. Both right and left colons are mobilized by lateral peritoneal incisions and these are extended along the iliac vessels and across the dome of the bladder to encompass all peritoneal tumor studding. The right colon is freely mobilized and the segment of cecum and terminal ileum to be resected is identified. The right colon, terminal mesentery, and small intestine are then transsected and the involved loops closed and pushed into the pelvis; an ileo-right colostomy is performed. Both ureters are identified retroperitoneally, and the entire pelvic peritoneum is swept medially and stripped from the posterior wall of the bladder. The uterine and vesical arteries may be transsected just medial to the ureters as dissection proceeds along them, or these vessels may be divided lateral to the ureters against the pelvic wall, the ureters later being teased from the side of the pelvic mass. They are rarely invaded, and usually do not need to be resected, the observed hydronephrosis being due to compression. The vaginal cuff is identified and the upper vagina is cross clamped and transsected below the clamp. The specimen is now held within the pelvis by the rectal stump, which is divided below the level of the cul-de-sac so that the entire pelvic peritoneum is removed. The sigmoid is transsected above the tumor mass and the specimen is removed, a primary colon anastomosis being performed. The ureters are held beneath the areolar tissue of the lateral pelvic wall with fine catgut sutures. Sump drainage is used within the pelvis.

Figure 5 demonstrates the effect of different treatment regimens on Stage IV ovarian cancers. The only long-term survivor at the Ellis Fischel Hospital had an abdominal wall implant resected with a locally advanced pelvic lesion, followed by irradiation. The use of irradiation after oophorectomy appeared to prolong survival.

Radiation therapy. Decision to administer radiotherapy should also be based on histology as well as stage of disease. LONG and associates in 1967 [8] reported 80 patients with ovarian cancer subjected to pelvic irradiation (table I). Granulosa carcinoma was the most responsive tumor with papillary, solid adenocarcinoma, and undifferentiated carcinoma following in that order. Dysgerminomas are also known to be quite radiosensitive. Mucinous tumors respond but rarely. KENT and MCKAY [5] also concluded that pseudomucinous tumors showed no radiation response. Of three patients with pseudomyxoma peritonei, none responded to radiation therapy [9].

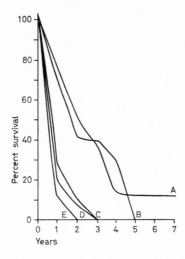

Fig. 5. Survival of patients with Stage IV carcinoma by method of treatment. A = wide hysterectomy and radiotherapy (8 patients); B = oophorectomy and radiotherapy (10 patients); C = oophorectomy alone (18 patients); D = no treatment (45 patients); E = radiotherapy alone (8 patients).

Table I. Rate of response of ovarian tumors to external radiotherapy with 220 kV or Co-60 equipment. Only those patients receiving an estimated tumor dose of 2,000 rads or more are included

Histologic type	No. treated	% eval. cases responding
Granulosa	3	100
Papillary	41	62.8
Adenocarcinoma	20	44.5
Unclassified carcinoma	5	33.0
Mucinous	10	16.0
Epidermoid	1	0
Total or average	80	51.0

Adjunctive radiotherapy cannot be justified for Stage I lesions considering the excellent survival obtained by surgical excision alone. Its greatest value is in the treatment of advanced stages. LONG and SALA [7] in 1963 reported eight patients with locally advanced ovarian cancer managed by irradiation followed by surgical resection. Only one patient in this series died, of intestinal fistulae, during a follow-up period up to 8 years. The 5-year survival rate was 100%. Four patients with Stage III cancer who received postoperative irradiation had a five year survival rate of 50%. Of four patients in this stage who had a radical procedure without irradiation, three died of recurrent cancer. BAER [1] in 1940 reported the regression of locally advanced ovarian carcinoma following X-ray therapy to an operable state. After excision of the uterus and adnexae, the patient was a 'long-term survivor'. PARKS [13] in 1945 reported three cases of locally advanced ovarian carcinoma managed by irradiation with subsequent resection, after preliminary laparotomy revealed an advanced inoperable state. CORSCADEN [3] later reported six cases of locally advanced ovarian lesions which were so managed. Four of these proved to be disease-free survivors.

Of patients with untreated Stage III tumors there are no survivors at five years. Surgical resection alone results in an extremely low survival. In the series reported by MUNNELL [11] adjunctive irradiation afforded a much greater survival in the advanced stages but this was not true for tumors confined to the ovaries, where a definitive surgical procedure alone resulted in a high percentage of cures. WALTER et al. [17] noted improvement in survival for all stages with adjunctive irradiation, but this was much less marked for Stages I and II and was particularly significant in Stages III and IV. KENT et al. [5] reported improvement in survival rates of all stages with added irradiation, but their results with surgical excision alone in Stages I and II seem low. It appears that pre-operative irradiation would be a method of choice in the care of Stage III tumors. For Stage IV (metastatic) lesions adjunctive irradiation appears to significantly influence duration of survival. RUBIN [14] reviewed the results of treatment with intraabdominal radioactive isotopes. While 52% of patients were improved, the ascites was controlled in only 5%.

Pseudomyxoma peritonei. This condition is discussed separately because its histology and response to irradiation and chemotherapy place it in an unusual category when compared to other advanced lesions. It may be derived from low grade mucin secreting tumors of the appendix or ovary. In the vast majority of these lesions the epithelium appears benign, although it is implanted throughout the peritoneal cavity. The abdomen is frequently distended by a large volume of gelatinous mucin, whose gross appearance is diagnostic of the condition. When untreated these patients die of intestinal obstruction. Recent experience has demonstrated that removal of the female pelvic viscera and appendix, as well as the complete evacuation of all mucin, with peritoneal washing and instillation of alkylating agents results in significantly increased asymptomatic survival (fig. 6). Oral estrogen therapy has been observed to induce objective and subjective improvement [9]. These tumors have consistently demonstrated a lack of response to irradiation. Operative intervention should be used to relieve intestinal obstruction when it occurs, as these patients do not develop solid tumor masses within the peritoneal cavity, and metastases beyond this area will not occur.

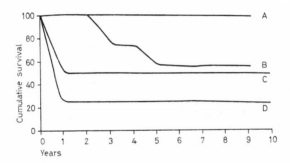

Fig. 6. Survival for patients with pseudomyxoma peritonei after initial treatment, comparing various treatment regimens. A = multiple operative procedure combined with alkylating agents (7 patients); B = multiple operative procedures (5 patients); C = paracentesis only (2 patients); D = oophorectomy or exploratory laparotomy only (5 patients).

Chemotherapy. Ovarian cancer has been responsive to chemotherapy with alkylating agents, with response rates varying from 40% to 50%. Thio-TEPA, chlorambucil, and phenylalanine mustard appear to be drugs of choice [4, 10]. RUTLEDGE and BURNS [15] have recently reported results with Stage IV cancers which are encouraging. They administered phenylalanine mustard to 288 patients. Of those who were observed six months or more, 123 responded and 36 did not. The most superior survival rates were obtained in those who received PAM first, followed by radiotherapy. It also appears that the rate of response is better in those patients who had their ovaries removed rather than a simple biopsy. Three courses of therapy, with a 3-

to 4-week interval between courses were attempted, using leukocyte or platelet counts for evaluation of bone marrow depression.

MASTERSON [10] has reported 19 survivors in over 300 patients with disseminated ovarian cancer treated on a chronic basis with chlorambucil. These patients received 0.2 mg per kg of body weight daily, divided into three equal postprandial portions. The drug was administered for three weeks with a rest of two weeks, the leukocyte count falling within the range of 1,500 to 4,000 cells/mm³. This course of therapy is given repeatedly, as long as the patient is able to tolerate therapy. Sixty per cent of patients so treated have responded, and one-quarter of these have been kept in remission for 2 years or more. MASTERSON also refers to patients with inoperable disease initially, who became operable after chemotherapy and were resected.

With extensive mucinous tumors, intraperitoneal administration of alkylating agents after resection of all tumor masses and evacuation of all gross mucin appears to provide extended symptom free survival. This may be repeated if the ascites recurs, or if celiotomy is again necessary for intestinal obstruction [9].

Hormonal therapy of tumors of the gonads remains largely unexplored [6]. Estrogen therapy appears clinically to benefit post-menopausal patients with pseudomyxoma of ovarian origin [9]. Ablation of ovarian function may be of value with low grade papillary lesions. The influence of adrenal function on such tumors has not been reported.

References

1. BAER, J. L.: in Discussion; in PEMBERTON Carcinoma of the ovary. Amer. J. Obstet. Gynec. 40: 751 (1940).
2. BARNES, P. H.: Oophorectomy in primary carcinoma confined to one ovary. Canad. med. Ass. J. 79: 416 (1958).
3. CORSCADEN, J. A.: Gynecologic cancer (Williams and Wilkins, Baltimore 1962).
4. HRESCHYSHYN, M. M. and HOLLAND, J. F.: Chemotherapy in patients with gynecologic cancer. Amer. J. Obstet. Gynec. 83: 468 (1962).
5. KENT, S. W. and McKAY, D. G.: Primary cancer of the ovary. Amer. J. Obstet. Gynec. 80: 430 (1960).
6. LONG, R. T. L. and EVANS, A. M.: Diethylstilbestrol as a chemotherapeutic agent for ovarian carcinoma. Missouri Med.: 1,125 (1963).
7. LONG, R. T. L. and SALA J. M.: Radical surgery combined with radiotherapy in the treatment of advanced ovarian carcinoma. Surg. Gyn. Obstet. 117: 201 (1963).

8. Long, R. T. L.; Johnson, R. E., and Sala, J. M.: Variations in survival among patients with ovarian carcinoma. Cancer 20: 1,195 (1967).
9. Long, R. T. L.; Spratt, J. S., and Dowling, E.: Pseudomyxoma peritonei; new concepts in therapy. Amer. J. Surg. 117: 162 (1969).
10. Masterson, J. G.: Tumor conference. Illinois med. J. 133: 410 (1968).
11. Munnell, E. W.; Jacox, H. W., and Taylor, H. C., Jr.: Treatment and prognosis in cancer of the ovary. Amer. J. Obstet. Gynec. 74: 1,187 (1957).
12. Pankamaa, P.: Pseudomyxoma pertonei. Acta chir. gynec. fenn., Supplement 74 47: 1 (1958).
13. Parks, T. J.: Carcinoma of the ovary treated postoperatively with deep X-ray; report of three cases. Amer. J. Obstet. Gynec. 49: 676 (1945).
14. Rubin, P.: A critical analysis of current therapy of carcinoma of the ovary. Amer. J. Roentgenol. 88: 833 (1962).
15. Rutledge, F. and Burns, B. C.: Chemotherapy for advanced ovarian cancer. Amer. J. Obstet. Gynec. 96: 761 (1966).
16. Van Orden, D. E.; McAllister, W. B., and Morris, G. M.: Ovarian carcinoma; the problems of staging and grading. Amer. J. Obstet. Gynec. 94: 195 (1966).
17. Walter, R. I.; Bachman, A. L., and Harris, W.: The treatment of carcinoma of the ovary- Improvement of results with postoperative radiotherapy. Amer. J. Roentgenol. 45: 403 (1941).

Author's address: Dr. Robert T. L. Long, 226 West Tennessee Street, Florence, AL 35630 (USA).

Front. Radiation Ther. Onc., vol. 5, pp. 262–275
(Karger, Basel/München/Paris/New York 1970)

Adenocarcinoma of the Uterus[1]

G. H. FLETCHER, F. N. RUTLEDGE, and L. DELCLOS

Department of Radiotherapy, The University of Texas M. D. Anderson Hospital and Tumor
Institute at Houston, Houston, Tex.

Introduction

Adenocarcinoma of the uterus can be found after fractional curettage to be limited to the endometrium or the uterine cervix, or to involve both, the so-called corpus et collum according to HEYMAN's terminology [14, 17]. The corpus et collum cases are Stage II endometrium of the FIGO classification.

There are three clinical situations which can be outlined for disease of the endometrium, corpus et collum, and cervix: (1) patients with operable lesions and good surgical risks, (2) patients with technically operable lesions but poor surgical risks, and (3) patients with disease too advanced for surgical resection. This essay will be limited to the treatment techniques and results in patients who are good surgical risk with a resectable lesion.

Cervix Only

As a rule, adenocarcinomas of the cervix are of endocervical origin. They commonly invade the myometrium and may grow to large lesions at the level of the endocervix and isthmus. This pattern of local growth allows them to remain longer in Stage I and II than do the squamous cell carcinomas. The tissues of the bladder, rectum, and ureters are more apt to be pushed aside by the

[1] This investigation was supported by Public Health Service Research Grants No. CA-06294 and CA-05654 from the National Cancer Institute.

expanding growth, rather than being incorporated into the cancer as with squamous cell carcinoma.

The primary radiotherapeutic management of adenocarcinomas limited to the cervix is that of the squamous cell carcinomas. Because of a lesser probability of lymphatic spread, there is a tendency to accentuate local radium therapy and de-emphasize external irradiation. For example, in a Stage II$_B$ lesion, only 2,000 rads may be delivered to the whole pelvis while radium would be correspondingly increased. Table I summarizes treatment planning.

The hysterectomy is conservative; the uterus is removed without an additional vaginal cuff, with minimum dissection of the bladder, ureters, and rectosigmoid colon. As much tissue as possible is removed with the cervix, without dissecting the ureters from their paracervical position. The conservative procedure has few complications and should be adequate to remove any residual cancer remaining within the myometrium. The procedure supplements the irradiation which gives an adequate dose to the vaginal mucosa and the paracervical area, but which may be somewhat inadequate in reaching cancer cells deep in the myometrium.

Corpus et collum

Because the spread to the vagina and the parametria is similar to that of adenocarcinoma of the cervix, intracavitary radium therapy is of the same type as that for squamous cell carcinoma of the

Table I. Adenocarcinoma of the cervix

Clinical situations	Treatment
Stage I and II Small lesion	Treat like squamous cell carcinoma Radium 2 applications for 72 h[1] 2 weeks apart ? Parametrial irradiation
Stage I and II Large central lesion	Add postradiation hysterectomy 4,000 rads whole pelvis One radium application – 72 h[1] Hysterectomy 4–6 weeks postradiation

[1] FLETCHER [11].

cervix. The Heyman packing technique is not used preoperatively but instead a tandem is used to give maximum paracervical irradiation in combination with the same type of vaginal radium therapy used for squamous cell carcinomas.

Whole pelvis irradiation is emphasized for large uteri and/or anaplastic tumors because the chances are greater that the tumor will reach the serosal surface of the uterus. Table II shows treatment techniques.

Table II. Adenocarcinoma of the corpus and cervix

Clinical situations	Treatment

Small or normal uterine cavity	Intracavitary radium
	    Tandem and colpostats – 72 h and 48 h applications
	    (like squamous cell carcinoma of cervix)[1] 2 weeks apart
	? Parametrial irradiation
	Hysterectomy, 4–6 weeks

Enlarged uterine cavity, no extension beyond uterus or cervix	4,000 rads whole pelvis
	Intracavitary radium
	    Tandem and colpostats – 72 h
	    (like squamous cell carcinoma of cervix)[1]
	Hysterectomy, 4–6 weeks

[1] FLETCHER [11].

Endometrium

Microscopic Pattern of Cancer of the Endometrium

In some endometrial carcinomas, the reproduction of the endometrial glands is so complete that the tissue is quite similar to benign endometrium and is described as a well-differentiated tumor. At the other extreme, only single cells or fragments of glands suggestive of the mother structure are present; this is described as a poorly differentiated tumor. In even more severe degrees of undifferentiation, the microscopic appearance is so amorphous that the tumor cannot be distinguished from sarcoma. When the cell type is one which apparently stems from the stroma of the endometrium, the diagnosis of sarcoma can be accurately made. In approximately 15% of the very poorly differentiated tumors, the pathologist has difficulty distinguishing adenocarcinoma from sarcoma.

Spread into the Myometrium

GUSBERG has observed that in tumors with a high degree of differentiation, myometrial invasion was only present in 20%, whereas in Grade III tumors, it was present in more than half of the cases [12].

Spread to the Vagina

Vaginal metastases present when the patient is first seen, as a rule, indicate widespread disease [19]. A 10 to 15% incidence of later spread to the vagina, mostly in the upper third, is reported in many series [3, 12, 13]. The mechanism of this spread is unknown.

Spread to Pelvic Structure

Spread to the broad ligaments, the fallopian tubes, and the ovaries is common. Excision of these tissues is a necessary part of the surgical procedure. The frequency of occurrence of these metastases is too great to allow preservation of the ovaries even when the patient is not of menopausal age.

Preoperative irradiation

When the uterus is of normal size and the tumor well differentiated, preoperative irradiation is probably of no value [13].

Intracavitary radium in the uterus and the vagina [1, 3, 4, 15], external irradiation alone [18, 21], and a combination of both [7] have seemingly achieved equal survival rates and prevented vaginal recurrences.

With the more anaplastic tumors and/or an enlarged uterus, one should emphasize whole pelvis irradiation. In the poorly differentiated carcinomas resembling sarcomas and the mixed mesodermal tumor, whole pelvis irradiation to at least 4,000 rads is given first.

Table III summarizes the policies of treatment and details of technique.

Table III. Adenocarcinoma of the endometrium technically and medically operable

Clinical situations	Treatment to uterus	Treatment to vagina
Small uterine cavity well differentiated tumor	Hysterectomy only	Wide vaginal cuff

Slightly enlarged uterine cavity, well differentiated tumor	Radium
	  1 – 72 h tandem or 3,000–
	  3,500 mg/h with packing
	Hysterectomy
		Colpostats
		  6,000 rads surface dose
		  in one application

Moderately enlarged uterine cavity (6–8 weeks size) well differentiated tumor	Radium
	  2,000 mg/h×2–3 weeks apart
	or
	4,000 rads whole pelvis and radium
	1 Heyman packing 2,500 mg/h or
	tandem 72 h with 15 and 10 mg sources
	Hysterectomy
		Colpostats
		  4,000 rads surface dose ×2
		  3 weeks apart
		  4,000 rads surface dose
		  1 application

Large uterine cavity or anaplastic tumor	4,000 rads whole pelvis and radium
	1 Heyman packing 2,500 mg/h or
	tandem 72 h with 15 and 10 mg sources
	Hysterectomy
		Colpostats
		  4,000 rads surface dose
		  1 application

The intrauterine γ-ray therapy can be applied with a tandem, if the uterine cavity shows no gross irregularity and the uterus is of normal size, in one insertion of 72 hours. In recent years, the Heyman's packing technique has been improved by adding an afterloading tandem (fig. 1) instead of a larger capsule placed in the endocervix. This allows one to choose the necessary radium to irradiate the lower uterine segment more adequately. Furthermore, the addition of the tandem, used as a lever, decreases severe anteflexion or retroflexion, reducing unnecessary high doses to the base of the bladder or rectum.

If 4,000 rads whole pelvis has been given, the No. 1 capsules are loaded with 5 mg radium tubes; the exposure to the personnel involved in the procedure is reduced to half and it is easier to match the time the capsules are left in place to deliver the vaginal surface dose from the colpostats which is aimed at 4,000 rads for each insertion.

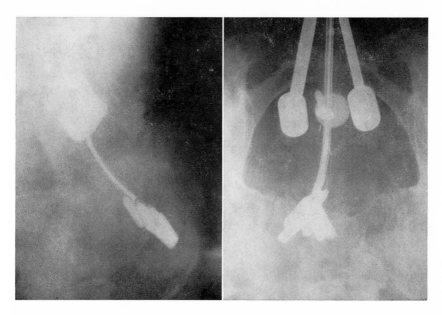

Fig. 1. Heyman packing with afterloading tandem. The use of an afterloading tandem in addition to the Heyman capsules allows a better irradiation of the endocervical canal. In addition, by using the rigid tandem as a lever one decreases severes anteflexion or retroflexion, and so reduces unnecessary high doses to the base of the bladder or rectum. The tandem is loaded as required for a better irradiation of the endocervix and paracervical area (for instance 5-5-15 when No. 1 capsules with 5 mg each are used, or 10-10-15 when No. 2 capsules with 10 mg each are used). The use of the afterloading colpostats or vaginal afterloading cylinders as indicated allows one to determine appropriate radium sources for a desired surface dose.

2,500 mg/h of radium are given twice in the uterine cavity, three weeks apart. If there is a question about performing a hysterectomy because of the patient's poor general condition, the dose is increased to 3,000 mg/h twice, also 3 weeks apart.

Vaginal radium is an important part of preoperative irradiation. Most vaginal recurrences develop on the vault and seldom develop in the lower third of the vagina [3, 9, 19]. Only colpostats are used or, in case of narrow vagina, a small vaginal cylinder. If possible, the colpostat applications are carried out at the time of the Heyman's packings with a total surface dose of approximately 8,000 rads. If the vagina is narrow, the application is done at one time between the two Heyman's packings with 6,000 to 7,000 rads surface dose given in 72 to 96 hours.

Operative findings

The operative findings are shown in table IV. Disease has been found in the pelvic structures (*i.e.,* ovaries, tubes, and peritoneal surface of the pelvic cavity) in 7% of the patients with endometrial cancer. In only one of 66 lymphadenectomies were nodes found to contain cancer (this patient also had tumor in the pelvic structures). This low incidence of involved regional nodes is not due to the previous irradiation because intracavitary radium alone, used in most patients, contributes little radiation to the regional lymphatics.

Six per cent of the patients with corpus et collum cancer had the pelvic structures involved, primarily the result of implants on the serosal surface of the uterus or pelvic organs, with local lesions apparently of small size. The incidence of positive involvement of regional and para-aortic nodes is 7% which is higher than for the endometrial group. This low incidence partially may result from external irradiation which was given either in the form of parametrial or whole pelvis irradiation.

Table IV. Operative findings (irradiation and surgery) adenocarcinoma of the uterus 1948 through December 1964

	Endometrium		Corpus et collum		Cervix, stages I and II	
	Number of patients	Dead of tumor	Number of patients	Dead of tumor	Number of patients	Dead of tumor
Negative uterus	145	6	35	2	28	1
Positive uterus only	69	7	33	5	26	5
Positive regional lymphatics only	0	0	5	3	1	1
Positive pelvic structures [1]	13 [2]	6	4	3	0	0
Positive paraaortic nodes	6 [3]	5	5 [4]	5	2	2 [5]
Totals	233	24	82	18	57	9

  [1] Tubes, ovaries, peritoneal surface of pelvic walls bladder, rectum and sigmoid.
  [2] One also had regional nodes.
  [3] Three also had pelvic disease.
  [4] One had pelvic disease and one had regional nodes also.
  [5] One also had regional nodes.

Courtesy: DELCLOS *et al.* [8].

The incidence of positive nodes in adenocarcinoma of the cervix only is low (2 of 57 patients had positive regional nodes; one of the 2 also had positive para-aortic nodes). Here again, external irradiation often having been given in many instances may be partially responsible for the low incidence of positive nodes; however, it seems that adenocarcinoma of the cervix does not spread as often to the regional lymphatics as does squamous cell carcinoma. Pelvic structures were not found to be involved.

The relatively high incidence of involvement of the para-aortic nodes without involvement of the regional lymphatics can be explained on the basis that the primary lymphatics of the corpus drain upward via the infundibulopelvic ligament. Thus, the first group of nodes encountered are the common iliac, lumbar, and para-aortic clusters.

Involvement of pelvic structures can perhaps be explained by tumor invading the myometrium and spreading through the serosa and/or through the fallopian tubes to the abdominal cavity.

Survival Rates and Sites of Failure

Table V shows the survival rates for patients with disease in the three anatomical locations. The patients with adenoacanthoma have the same survival rate as those with adenocarcinoma exhibiting a similar clinical behavior [2].

Table V. Five-year absolute survival rates adenocarcinoma of the uterus (previously untreated patients), resectable lesions in good medical risk patients 1948 through December 1962

Endometrium	Corpus et collum	Cervix Stage I		Stage II	
		Irrad.	Irrad.+surg.	Irrad.	Irrad.+surg.
144/181 (79%)	36/61 (59%)	7/8	10/11	7/13	12/16

For the lesions limited to the cervix, the survival rates are equally as good as for squamous cell carcinoma [20]. There is no evidence in Stage I cases that the addition of hysterectomy is of benefit but despite the small numbers there is the suggestion that additional hysterectomy is worthwhile in Stage II cases. If no lymphadenectomy is performed, the complications of conservative hysterectomy are minimal. Therefore, when one deals with an endocervical and somewhat bulky lesion, the uncertainty of how much of the myometrium is involved justifies adding conservative hysterectomy to the plan of treatment to increase its effectiveness.

The results in corpus et collum cases are not as good as are those in patients with disease limited to the endometrium or the cervix [8].

Concerning the endometrial cancers, review of the undifferentiated tumors [10] clearly showed better survival rates when preoperative irradiation was given (table VI). Also Table VI shows that for the separate group of mixed mesodermal sarcomas survival rates were superior when preoperative irradiation was used [10]. It is of interest that there were instances of tumor sterilization in the operative specimen of mixed mesodermal sarcomas.

A review of the sites of failures for the technically operable cases shows that pelvic failures were about the same in the three groups. Distant metastases are the main cause of death of patients with tumors of the corpus et collum.

Table VI. Five-Year absolute survival rates

No. of patients alive/No. of patients treated			
Undifferentiated tumors		Mixed mesodermal sarcomas	
No preop. irrad.	Preop. irrad.	No preop. irrad.	Preop. irrad.
6/21[1]	15/29[1]	2/13[1]	9/21[1]

[1] In both cases the trend is in favor of the preoperative irradiation but the number of patients is too small to establish statistical significance.

Vaginal metastases are rare after preoperative irradiation [5, 6, 9, 12, 16, 18, 19] which is also confirmed in our material (table VII). To prevent vaginal recurrences, it is not necessary to treat the whole vagina, since in the M. D. Anderson Hospital material, as in other series [9] observed recurrences are primarily on the vault. Recurrences are rarely solitary but are but one manifestation of diffuse spread.

Table VII. Vaginal recurrences correlated to vaginal radium modalities (preoperative group endometrial cancers), September 1948–December 1960

Site		Colpostats[2] cylinder[1]	Bloedorn[2] applicator	Colpostats Only[3]	Misc. techniques	No vaginal radium
Number of patients		34	67	77	7	3
Vault	0					
Lower 1/3 vagina	1		1			
Vault[2] pelvis	1			1		
Vault, pelvis distant metastases	4		1	2		1

5 of 185 patients treated (2.7%).

[1] 1st insertion — 4,000 rads/vault (ovoids);
2nd insertion — 4,000 rads/whole vagina (cylinder).   total vault dose 8,000 rads
[2] 1 insertion — 7,000 rads/whole vagina.
[3] 2 insertions — 4,000 rads/vault each insertion.

Courtesy: DELCLOS and FLETCHER [7].

Summary

Hysterectomy after irradiation is performed routinely in the management of patients with resectable adenocarcinoma of the endometrium and corpus et collum who are considered to be good surgical risk but not systematically for Stages I and II adenocarcinoma of the cervix. Preoperative irradiation techniques vary with the site of origin, the extent of involvement, and the histology of the tumor.

References

1. ARNESON, A. N.: Long term follow-up observations in corporeal cancer. Amer. J. Roentgenol. *91:* 3–21 (1964).

2. BORONOW, R. C.: Carcinoma of the corpus; in Cancer of the uterus and ovary, a collection of papers presented at the 11th Annual Clinical Conference on Cancer, 1966, at the University of Texas M. D. Anderson Hospital and Tumor Institute at Houston, Texas, pp. 35–61 (Year Book, Medical Publishers, Inc., Chicago 1969).

3. CHAU, P. M.: Technic and evaluation of preoperative radium therapy in adenocarcinoma of the uterine corpus; in Carcinoma of the uterine cervix, endometrium and ovary. A Collection of Papers Presented at the 5th Annual Clinical Conference on Cancer, 1960, at The University of Texas M. D. Anderson Hospital and Tumor Institute at Houston, Texas, pp. 235–256 (Year Book, Medical Publishers, Inc., Chicago 1962).

4. COSTOLOW, W. E.; NOLAN, J. F.; BUDENZ, G. C., and DuSAULT, L.: Radiation treatment of carcinoma of the corpus uteri. Amer. J. Roentgenol. *71:* 669–675 (1954).

5. DOBBIE, M. W.: Vaginal recurrences in carcinoma of the body of the uterus and their prevention by radium therapy. J. Obstet. Gynaec. Brit. Cwlth. *60:* 702–705 (1953).

6. DAVIS, E. W. Jr.: Carcinoma of the corpus uteri. Amer. J. Obstet. Gynec. *88:* 163–170 (1964).

7. DELCLOS, L. and FLETCHER, G. H.: Malignant tumors of the endometrium. Evaluation of some aspects of radiotherapy; in cancer of the uterus and ovary, a collection of papers presented at the 11th Annual Clinical Conference on Cancer, 1966, at The University of Texas M. D. Anderson Hospital and Tumor Institute at Houston, Texas, pp. 62–72 (Year Book, Medical Publishers, Inc., Chicago 1969).

8. DELCLOS, L.; FLETCHER, G. H.; GUTIERREZ, A. G., and RUTLEDGE, F. N.: Adenocarcinoma of the uterus. Amer. J. Roentgenol. *105:* 603–608 (1969).

9. DOUGLAS, R. G.: Personal commun (1964).

10. EDWARDS, C. L.: Undifferentiated tumors; in Cancer of the uterus and ovary, a collection of papers presented at the 11th Annual Clinical Conference on Cancer, 1966, at The University of Texas M. D. Anderson Hospital and Tumor Institute at Houston, Texas, pp. 84–94 (Year Book, Medical Publishers, Inc., Chicago 1969).

11. FLETCHER, G. H.: Uterine cervix; in Textbook of radiotherapy, pp. 440–456 (Lea & Febiger, Philadelphia 1966).

12. GUSBERG, S. B.; JONES, H. C. Jr., and TOVELL, H. M. M.: Selection of treatment for corpus cancer. Amer. J. Obstet. Gynec. *80:* 374–380 (1960).

13. GUSBERG, S. B. and YANNOPOULOS, D.: Therapeutic decisions in corpus cancer. Amer. J. Obstet. Gynec. *88:* 157–162 (1964).

14. HEYMAN, J.; REUTERWALL, O., and BENNER, S.: The Radiumhemmet experience with radiotherapy in cancer of the corpus of the uterus. Acta radiol., Stockh. *22:* 11–98 (1941).

15. HUNT, H. B.: Comparative radiotherapeutic results in carcinoma of the endometrium as modified by prior surgery and postirradiation hysterosalpingo-oophorectomy. Radiology *66:* 653–666 (1956).

16. INGERSOLL, F. M. and MEIGS, J. V.: Lymph node dissection for carcinoma of the endometrium; in Proc. Sec. Nat. Cancer Conf., vol. 1, pp. 747–752 (American Cancer Society, New York 1952).

17. KOTTMEIER, H.-L.: Carcinoma of the corpus. Its classification and treatment. Gynaecologia *138:* 287–310 (1954).

18. LAMPE, I.: Endometrial carcinoma. Amer. J. Roentgenol., *90:* 1,011–1,015 (1963).

19. RUTLEDGE, F. N.; TAN, S. K., and FLETCHER, G. H.: Vaginal metastases from adenocarcinoma of the corpus uteri. Amer. J. Obstet. Gynec. *75:* 167–174 (1958).

20. RUTLEDGE, F. N.; GUTIERREZ, A., and FLETCHER, G. H.: Management of Stage I and II adenocarcinoma of the uterine cervix on intact uterus. Amer. J. Roentgenol. *102:* 161–164 (1968).
21. SALA, J. M. and DEL REGATO, J. A.: Treatment of carcinoma of the endometrium. Radiology *79:* 12–17 (1962).

Authors' addresses: Dr. GILBERT H. FLETCHER, Head, Department of Radiotherapy, The University of Texas, M. D. Anderson Hospital and Tumor Institute, *Houston, TX 77025;* Dr. FELIX N. RUTLEDGE, Chief, Gynecology Service, Department of Surgery, The University of Texas, M. D. Anderson Hospital and Tumor Institute, *Houston, TX 77025* (USA); Dr. LUIS DELCLOS, Radiotherapist, Hospital General de Asturias, *Oviedo* (Spain).

Discussion

Moderator:

K. WARREN NEWGARD, M. D., Associate Clinical Professor of Obstetrics and Gynecology, University of California Medical Center, San Francisco, Calif.

Discussant:

FRANZ J. BUSCHKE, M.D., Professor of Radiology; Chief, Section of Therapeutic Radiology, University of California Medical Center, *San Francisco, Calif.*

BUSCHKE: I want to emphasize mainly one point with regard to the treatment of ovarian papillary adenocarcinoma that has become more and more obvious to us during the last years, and should influence treatment really to a considerable degree. That is, that the extent of the disease, as long as it is limited to the abdomen, should not be a contraindication for treatment. I don't know any lesion as unpredictable as ovarian carcinoma, and I have patients considered hopeless who have made the grade.

One of them who particularly impressed me was seen back in 1940. She was a 28-year old woman with a frozen pelvis. The surgeon had reported that he scooped tumor out of the pelvis. The tumor disappeared completely under pelvic irradiation and the pelvis became perfectly normal. After five years she had on her routine examination an apparent recurrence of two masses which were movable and could be removed. Since then she has been recurrence free 29 years post-diagnosis. The microscopic material was repeatedly reviewed and the diagnosis confirmed. I have several cases of this kind.

What we have learned about them is, however, that we should not be satisfied when the pelvis becomes normal to palpation. That is the time when re-operation should be performed and all of the pelvic genital organs removed. We had some that have recurred after 5 or 6 years and became rapidly inoperable. I think it is important to keep in mind that in carcinoma of this type we think the best procedure is to explore them: If they are not frankly operable they should have as little surgery as possible, enough for biopsy, and staging and then should have radical radiation therapy. They should then be re-operated if the pelvic findings seem to justify it.

I would like to bring out one general point. We have undoubtedly now convinced the surgeons that radical surgery can be done after radical radiation therapy, if the radiation therapy is done with the surgery in mind and somewhat adjusted so the tissues are in good shape. Those surgeons who still object to it are usually the ones who have a lot of complications anyhow.

I would also like to reemphasize one sentence that Dr. GALANTE said here yesterday: 'The selection of the patients for this method of treatment cannot be scientifically infallible, as it is a subjective process that depends almost entirely on the clinical judgment and experience of the clinicians involved in this decision.' I think that for this reason, all the remarks made in these papers here have to be interpreted in this fashion. A scientific evaluation of this kind of combined procedure, including the randomized patient, seems to me impossible. It is a matter of individual decision in each patient. We should accept the fact that a team of equally competent members is needed. The factors that enter into such a decision are not only determined by the patient and his or her disease, but to a large degree by the philosophies and skills of the physicians working together. There are no fixed rules. Otherwise, this close cooperation necessary for such procedures cannot be achieved. In this light, this method does not differ really, to my mind, from other good clinical methods which have been in use since the time of Hippocrates. After all, medicine has never been a pure science, and there is always a subjective or artistic element concerned with it that we cannot entirely eliminate. I think this is even more true for this kind of joint approach than it is for many other methods in cancer therapy.

NEWGARD: We're using expressions, particularly the radiotherapists, that are somewhat loose from the point of view of the gynecologist. I should say more correctly, the gynecologists may misinterpret some of the statements made by the radiotherapists.

First is the 'fractionated curettage', one of the biggest problems for the pathologist. Most people using fractionated curettage just curette a little within the endocervical canal. I personally would like the procedure eliminated. In order to determine if there is extension to the endocervix, I would prefer taking a small gall bladder forceps, or any small biting instrument, and actually bite into the endocervix in order to find out if there is carcinoma in this tissue, attached to or invading the endocervical mucosa. What the pathologist most often gets, unfortunately, are loose pieces of tissue of adenocarcinoma. He has no idea if this material was lying free in the canal or actually coming from the endocervix.

Second is 'uterine size'. We are talking about large and small uteri. We should talk about large and small uterine *cavities* as measured with a sound, or ballooned-out uterine cavities, about smooth or irregular uterine cavities. Uterine 'size' changes with the age of the patient, with other pathologic states, and it is really not, as we use the term, the size of the 'uterus', but particularly the size of the cavity we are interested in. So we should be a little more specific in those terms.

Third is 'conservative hysterectomy'. The picture in gynecologic surgery has changed; today the conservative hysterectomy is considered the Richardson or intrafascial type of hysterectomy, which is not what Dr. FLETCHER means. Dr. FLETCHER means an *extra*fascial, or extended hysterectomy, as originally described by Wertheim, without node dissection. This operation leaves the uterosacral ligaments and the posterior leaves of the broad ligament untouched. In other words, the surgeon tries not to dislocate the ureters from their beds and still take adequate material, including the cervical fascia. This is not usually explained and we always hear talk about a 'conservative hysterectomy', which nobody really means.

I have one question for Dr. FLETCHER, and that is regarding your mesodermal tumors, with 50% survival. Did any of these cases have myometrial involvement, or were these all cases which were limited to the mucosa and were sterilized by X-ray? Your statistics are so much better than any others I know of.

FLETCHER: Dr. NEWGARD is making my life really difficult because I'm not qualified to answer most of those questions, but I will be glad to report to Dr. RUTLEDGE, our gynecologist, about the problems mentioned. Actually, we do mean large uterine cavities when we refer to a large uterus. The hysterectomy performed is not the one you do for fibroids, but an extrafascial one. You are correct in this terminology.

Concerning the mesodermal tumors, one-third of the patients who had preoperative irradiation had no disease left in the myometrium. The radioresistance of mixed mesodermal sarcoma is also a kind of myth. We have had through the years some mixed mesodermal sarcomas recurring in the vagina following hysterectomy. Some of these are very radio-